An intimate and moving account of the challenges and promise of contemporary family caregiving. This book provides practical advice and solutions to what is often a labyrinth of choices, problems, and barriers in the social/health care system. George and Emily Watson offer their heartfelt personal experiences so that others may gain courage and insight into the dynamics of caring for one's parents. I recommend this book to both family members and the professionals who work with them.

Scott D. Wright, Ph.D.
Gerontology Center
University of Utah

Readers of this highly personal account of caring for aging parents at the end of their lives can learn much. I especially appreciate three valuable insights that the Watsons share from their experiences. First, understanding that you can provide care is a source of empowerment. Those who desire to care for their dying parents need to know that they can do it. Second, there are alternatives to having your parents die in an institution such as a nursing home. The Watsons provide a splendid example of one alternative. Third, in an era when so much attention is given to the burden of elder care, it is refreshing to hear about personal rewards that can come from it. The insights into life and death and the fulfillment of meeting the needs that no one else can meet in the same way are tremendous. Hopefully many will benefit from this account of one couple's experiences.

Peter Uhlenberg, Ph.D.
Professor of Sociology
University of North Carolina, Chapel Hill

The Calling—A Journey on the Path of Parent Care is a wonderful book written from the perspectives of caregivers. This book is helpful for caregivers as it gives good advice and helps unravel some of the confusion and frustration when a person finds him/herself in the caregiving role. It is a must read for geriatric professionals as it reminds us of the human elements of the caregivers and care recipients that is often forgotten in the shuffle of paper work and large case loads.

Peter Hebertson
Program Manager
Salt Lake County Aging Services

This wonderful book is a unique combination of concise, accurate descriptions of aspects of "the system" and its hurdles, together with candid remarks about the joys and heartaches of family and close relationships. Anyone involved in caring for older people will benefit from reading about George and Emily's experiences, wisdom and emotions. The Calling truly moves forward, in a significant way, the work of elder care.

Karen M. Thomas, RN, BSN, JD
Registered Nurse, Licensed Attorney
Private Elder Law Practice
Salt Lake City, Utah

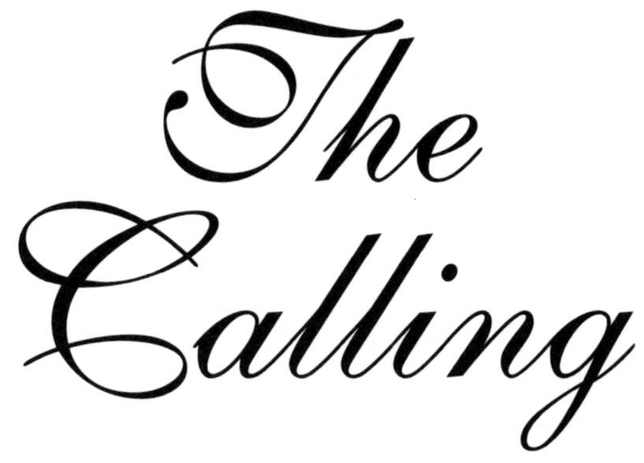

A Journey
on the Path
of
Parent Care

George & Emily Watson

The Calling
by George & Emily Watson

Author's note: The names of all private organizations have been altered to preserve confidentiality. Any similarity to organizations is purely coincidental.

For additional copies or for information regarding speaking engagements call:
(888) 380-8174

E-mail: gew@call-pmd.com

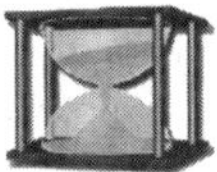

P M D, Inc.

Publisher's Cataloging-in-Publication
(Provided by Quality Books, Inc.)

Watson, George W.
The calling : a journey on the path of parent care / George & Emily Watson. -- 1st ed.
p. cm.
Includes index.
ISBN: 1-888106-90-5
LCCN: 97-077567

1. Parents, Aged--Care--United States. 2. Adult children--United States--Family relationships. 3. Caregivers--United States --Psychology. 4. Aged--Services for--United States. I. Watson, Emily A. II. Title.

HQ1063.6.W38 1998 649.8
QBI97-41346

Cover design Robert White
Cover Photo Linda Pettavino

Printed and bound
in the
United States of America
by

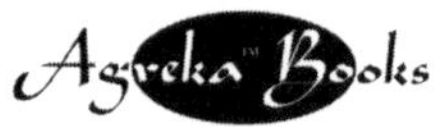

800 360-5284
www.agreka.com

The Calling

Our parents allowed us to walk with them through their late age journey to the door of death. It was a journey that was both humbling and enlightening. The final gift to us was insight we gained in sharing in their final years. We share this insight with all who embrace the challenge of parent care. As for this book, it is dedicated to the memories of our parents.

Table of Contents

Acknowledgments

We thank our editors Louis Roussalis, M.D., Amanda Pecor, Bob Donohoe, Nancy Bailey and William and Cynthia Grua for their endless support in our many revisions. Additional acknowledgments go to Home Health agencies, Hospice and nursing home staff who encouraged us in our goal of home care, the Senior Companion Program, Salt Lake Community Services' Chore and Assist, Salt Lake City Library Program, BOND, Michelle Hochberg of the Baltimore, Maryland Department of Health and Human Services for allowing us to incorporate the new sample Medicare forms, James Ziter, Beth Hanlon, M.D., Mary Jane Norman, M.D., Jeff Anderson, Alan Durtschi, Sue Lagman, Sandra Christensen, Eli Morales, Rose Anderton, Darrin Porter, Rudolph Murray, John Smith, Rudolpho Roca, Ken Rozema, Carol Smedley-Lucero, John McHugh, Nellie Stewart, Opal Stamper, Chris and Stephanie Dansie, The LDS Relief Society Ladies—Lucille Kerr & Lucy Bodily, Father Cassian for his prayers and Father Thomas for his sage advice, Evans and Early Mortuary of Salt Lake City, Utah, Fackler-Wiedeman Funeral Home, Harrisburg, Pennsylvania and Dickerson Funeral Home, Vanceburg, Kentucky. Our family support included Lloyd and Boots Cravens, Ella Hanger, Ruby Knight, Hazel Bradford, Joe and Bonnie Watson, Bob and Belle Watson, Byron & Barbara Watson, John Watson, Barbara Ensminger, Steve and Leslee Ensminger and Veronica Wolfe. The help of all these individuals contributed to our dedication in caring for our parents.

The omission of names is by no means a reflection of a lack of appreciation; every kind word, every dinner, dessert, flower or hour given to us by a neighbor or stranger deeply moved us, especially during difficult times. Successful in-home care truly does take a community and we will never forget how all of you in your own way walked this path with us.

Special Thanks

Mother Teresa wrote Emily,

> "You belong to a larger family. Jesus is the Vine and we are His branches. He sustains us with spiritual sap – with the grace that comes to us through the Sacraments . . . After receiving Him in the Bread of Life, you will reach out to Him in the suffering people – especially to your own who need your love and care."

A special thank you to Mother Teresa for teaching that we need not travel half way around the world to find people who are suffering.

Preface

By 2030 approximately 70 million people will be at least 65 years old. We need to prepare ourselves now so we will be ready for this geriatric population wave.

We decided to write this book because many of our friends, relatives and acquaintances, ill-prepared to care for their aging parents and loved ones, have come to us for advice. Between the two of us, we have had more than twenty years experience caring for our parents in residential and long-distance caregiving. Emily has had three years experience in nursing home and hospice care. We both graduated from the University of Utah's two year Gerontology certificate program and are state-certified Long-term Care Ombudsman with Salt Lake County Aging Services in Salt Lake City, Utah. As Ombudsman, we advocate for the rights of the elderly in long-term nursing and residential care facilities, investigate problems and help mediate solutions. We speak publicly to community groups on aging issues.

Today, major care is being provided in approximately seven million households in the United States and most of the people giving this care have had little or no training or experience. They lack the knowledge necessary to be good caregivers. Approximately eighty percent of all in-home care received by elderly people seventy-five or older is provided by family members. Caregivers who have full- or part-time jobs outside the home provide almost as many hours of care as do those who are not employed.

Successful caregiving can be accomplished under the most adverse circumstances. Even though we did not care for our parents while caring for children, we held down full-time jobs, tended to home maintenance on two homes and coped with chemotherapy: we both had cancer while caring for parents in our home.

Our experience has provided us with an opportunity to focus on the real issues of aging: preparing financially and learning to accept help graciously. Given our experience, we don't buy into the myth of ageism—that aging makes all people senile, unattractive, asexual, weak and useless. In observing our parents, we have seen quite the opposite can be true.

We hope sharing our stories will help you resolve many of the problems and frustrations that accompany elder caregiving. Should you choose to care for an elderly parent, you must learn all you can to be a part of the caregiving team which includes the caregiver, doctors, nurses, aides and therapists. Deciding to walk with our parents' on this part of their life's journey is the reason we attended the University of Utah Gerontology program and therapy sessions at a local rehabilitation center.

For those who question their obligation to care for their elderly parents, consider the following 600-year-old European folktale:

> A lonely widower struck a bargain with his son that he would be taken care of in his old age in return for turning over his property to the son while he was still alive. Later on, when the father became quite invalid, the daughter-in-law nagged her husband to move the old man to the barn. The son, ashamed to do it himself, had the grandson take the old man to the barn and wrap him with a horse blanket. The grandson tearfully obeyed his father, but ripped the horse blanket into two pieces and wrapped the old man in only half. When the father found out what his son had done, he became angry and demanded, "How could you be so cruel as to leave your grandfather in the barn to freeze with only half a blanket?" The son replied, "Father, I felt obligated to save the other half for you."

Whether your experience with parent care is in your own home or involves overseeing caregiving provided in a care facility, we feel you must take an active part in ensuring your parent's later life is safe and comfortable. We want to impress upon you that caring for your parents can be a time of enlightenment, fulfillment and closure. We hope our book will make caregiving much easier.

George and Emily Watson

Emily's Mother

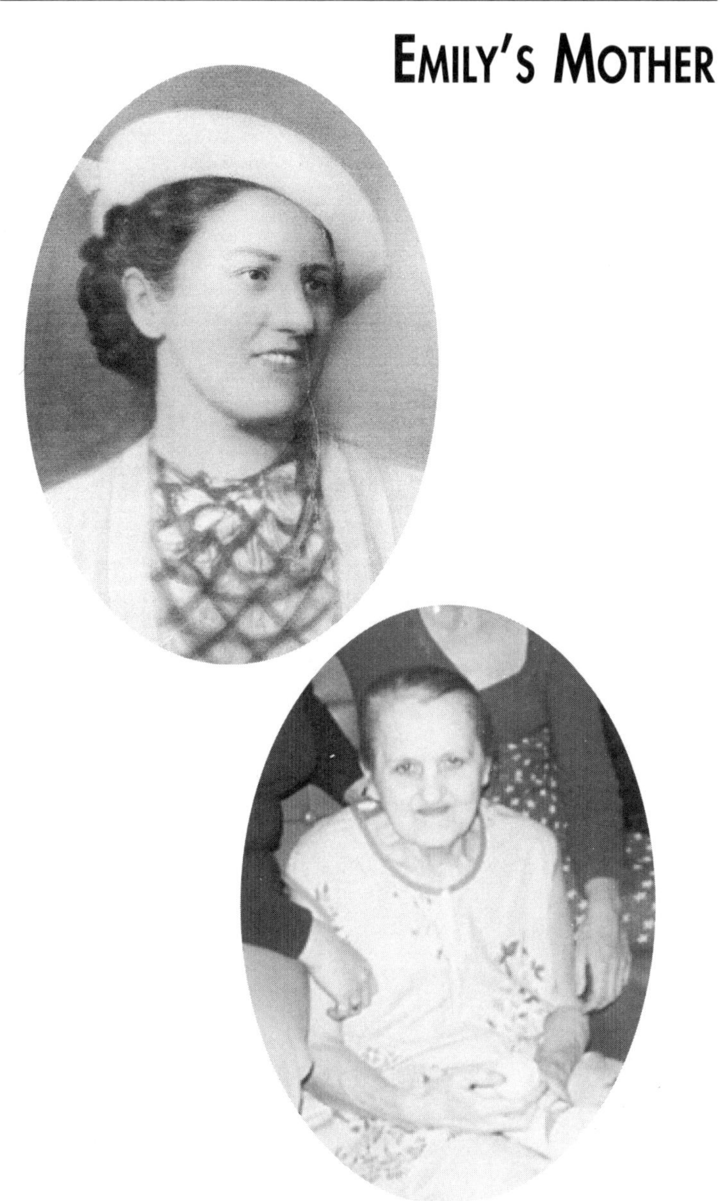

Elizabeth Alberta Kvaka Albert

August 18, 1912 — July 12, 1976

My earliest memory of my parents is shadowed by my mother's ill health and how it affected our household. We were a lower-middle-class family. The financial pressures, along with the patience and understanding required for Mother's care, produced frustrations and strong emotions.

Prior to my birth, Mother had been in and out of hospitals for various physical and emotional disorders due to what the doctors told us was a chemical imbalance. My father, in his attempts to keep order in the house, was controlling and domineering. Building a child's self-esteem was not part of his agenda—he didn't have the time or energy for that kind of parenting. Even if caring for my mother had been less overwhelming, I don't believe he would have known where to begin. I am the youngest of three girls and by the time I was ten years old, my two older sisters had moved out of the house and Dad's energy revolved around his work and coping with Mother. He had no time left over for me.

When I was fourteen, I had the opportunity to live abroad with my oldest sister and her family. My father encouraged this move because he felt he could not deal with me and my mother at the same time. Much to my father's relief and my mother's disbelief, I accepted the invitation. I finished school under my sister's supervision. During this time, I developed friendships with kids my father disapproved of because of their race. Eventually, my father disowned me. "You are no longer my daughter," he said.

As her daughters left home, Mother became more and more withdrawn. My father, now retired, found his home a lonely, loveless place where honoring his commitment to the marriage was an overwhelming burden.

Three years after I graduated from high school, my father, even with my middle sister's help, reached his limit in coping with Mother's illness. He was tired of caring for her, especially since she was now confined to a living room chair. Mother sensed how he felt toward her and was frightened. She asked me to come home, an experience that changed the course of my life.

I learned when my mother was dying that caring for a parent involves not only meeting his or her physical needs but also coming to terms with personal histories. It was only when I returned to my mother's side in her final days that I started down the road that would, at a much later date, lead me to make peace with the unresolved pain of my childhood.

Taking on the challenge of eldercare gave me the opportunity to make a positive difference in someone's life during a difficult transition, as well as a chance to face my transitions through aging and mortality. Eldercare could have the same effect for you.

Respecting the Rights of the Elderly

Sweat rolled down her face. She shifted and turned, hardly catching her breath as she suddenly awoke to the loud ticking of the clock. She sat on the edge of her chair, crying softly, biting the side of her finger, trying not to alert anyone to the fact that she was awake. She had come to a decision. I lay quietly on the other side of the room watching her stare in quiet anxiety. Soon she began to pray. "Hail Mary Full of Grace."

A month earlier Mom had been told, "If you don't have this operation your chances of living another three months are slim." Gangrene, a complication of her diabetes, had set in and would have killed her eventually. This was the situation facing my 63-year-old mother in 1976. Her decision was made only after many hours of talking, questioning and soul searching. The choice came down to how to live or how to die.

My mother weighed her options thoughtfully, thoroughly. If she agreed to have her leg amputated, she could move to California, where I lived and could care for her or she could spend the rest of her life in "the poor house" as my father so eloquently put it. She chose to let her diabetes take its course: she chose to die.

At that point the behavior of the medical professionals, clergy and family members took a major turn that was heartbreaking as well as disgusting. Instead of providing the support my mother desperately needed, her "support system" waged a battle against her choice. Medical professionals congregated in the kitchen with my father and plotted what to do with Mother. Then, as a group, they went into her room and told her about the plans they had made. When Mom turned to me with pleading eyes, I cleared the room so we could breath and consider what they had presented. She was terrified.

Based on the doctor's recommendation, my father tried to obtain a durable power of attorney. After all, they said, "She must be incompetent, because it's crazy to choose death." My father wanted to have control so he could authorize both the operation and her placement into the county nursing home; however, Dad needed my signature and I refused to sign. At that point, Mother and I were on our own and everyone washed their hands of us. The medical professionals and clergy focused their attention on my father's need to "get her out of the house." Father's pastor told Mother that if she agreed to go to the hospital peacefully he would send her a dozen red roses. When I heard this I became hysterical. But my mother and I could not alter the path of events. My mother was moved to the hospital, never to see her home again.

Once at the hospital, Mother had to focus on another difficult choice—where she would go to die. The two of us were at a loss until we met a hospice nurse named Joy. Hospice focuses on comfort measures to promote the quality of life for people who are dying, also referred to as *dying with dignity*. This concept has been embraced by numerous trained professionals who help people cope with death, either at home or in a facility.

Joy presented Mother with her options in nursing homes based on the family income and Mother chose one located in Hershey, Pennsylvania. Joy was sensitive and caring toward my mother during the transition from one "home" to another.

While I stood by Mother in her choice to die, I fought an internal battle to accept her surrender to death. I was disappointed she felt that to live as an amputee would be too much of an inconvenience for us. Even worse, I was disappointed in myself for not offering her a more acceptable option. I live with the thought that had I given up my job in California and moved back to Pennsylvania, she would have moved in with me and I could have cared for her. I never made that offer because I wasn't strong enough to face the past.

I listened as she said her good-byes to friends and relatives. She told me who to call and after I dialed that person's number she took the telephone from me and made her closure with the person right then. The most difficult phone call she asked me to make was the one to my father who had refused to visit her in the hospital. After dialing his number, I handed Mother the telephone and left the room. I remained outside of her door within earshot and I heard her say in a calm voice, "I want to make amends to you for all the trouble I've caused." I couldn't listen any longer so I left, feeling in awe of her, growing angry at my father for not initiating the call. Earlier that day Mother had asked me to forgive him. She also had tried to convince me that I should consider getting married, saying marriages didn't have to be what I had seen growing up. But I said "never" to both of her requests.

I realized my father had done what he thought was best. I realized my mother's advice to forgive was wise. Still for a number of years I remained resentful toward him. I rarely made contact. When I did it was only out of a sense of responsibility toward keeping in touch with my remaining parent.

It is important for dying people to take care of unfinished business. It is equally important for caregivers to resolve unfinished business between themselves and their elderly charges. Then caring for a parent can be a response to present circumstances and not a reaction to the past. Resolving personal affairs and negative emotions will free you later when your time to die is near. The adage, "What we resist, persists," is true. As you will see later in this book, I ultimately found myself in the position of facing my resentment toward my father.

When Mother was admitted to the nursing home, I returned to California to make arrangements for time off from work. The company agreed to transfer me to the Philadelphia office, which would put me near Mother until she died. I never made that move. I had been in California four days when I received a phone call from one of my sisters saying Mother wasn't expected to live through the week. I headed back East that night but Mother died while I was in flight.

My mother's experience is not unique. When we are old and our physical bodies break down, we may be faced with similar choices. What will our options be? Will we find the support we need? Will our right to make our own choices be respected? Will there be someone there for us to help us and truly speak on our behalf?

People who are frail want the same things we all want: safety, autonomy and a quality life. If we put ourselves in their shoes for a moment, we can see it is very difficult for them to live and die maintaining a sense of dignity. And while some things have changed, we must still become advocates for the elderly population or the time may come when we find ourselves *truly* in their shoes.

Sometimes caregivers, medical professionals and family assume the elderly cannot make decisions for themselves. These individuals then attempt to make life or death decisions on behalf of the ones they are caring for. When decisions are made based on assumptions, the rights of that person are violated.

I had the misfortune of witnessing this type of proprietary behavior during the months leading up to my mother's death. Who has the responsibility to ensure the rights of the elderly are respected? The responsibility belongs to all of us: family members, medical professionals, neighbors, church members and friends. We must all work to change attitudes toward the aged and work cooperatively to affirm the value of the human spirit so people of all ages are treated with dignity, especially when physical capabilities diminish during the dying process.

Interlude in Calcutta

After mother's death, I returned to California. During the next eighteen months I succumbed to a calling to work with the dying elderly through nursing homes and hospice. It was in this role—participating in the last days of people's life and witnessing their deaths—that I realized a deeper sense of people, of their beauty and of the spiritual walks we individually take.

During this period, I read of Mother Teresa and her work with destitute and dying people in India. I felt compelled to be in her presence and work with her. I sold what I had, adding the proceeds to my savings, quit my office job of eight years and started my new pursuit. I moved to Utah to be near my sister Barbara as I prepared to leave the country.

While in Utah, I wrote the Sisters of Charity in New York and Calcutta. I waited for their responses and applied for a work visa in India. I continued to work with the dying elderly in a Salt Lake City Nursing Home and through a hospice program. In Salt Lake City I met George (my husband to be) who, wise years ahead of me, was already tending to the needs of his parents on a part time basis. Our relationship grew. But my desire to learn from Mother Teresa and to work with her was still strong. It led me on to India in January of 1980. Feeling much like an excited carrier pigeon, I left the United States with gifts for Mother Teresa's work—food and money from people in Utah and chalices, ciborium and veils from nuns in Mother Teresa's order in New York.

Once I arrived at the Mother House and the gifts were delivered I began working with the missionaries. Walking through the streets of Calcutta on the way to the mission, I was amazed at how rich in spirit the "pavement dwellers" appeared to be. At times I felt like a spectator of life. I was in awe of what I saw.

After a two week interlude with this very special city and its people, I had the great fortune of spending time talking with the woman I had come to admire: a woman who reflected God's love in what she did and said. Her words to me were gentle but unwavering. Mother Teresa said, "The needs in India are food, shelter and clothes but your people don't know how to love and that is a much harder need to fulfill. You abandon your elderly and your babies. The work in your country is great."

My stay in Calcutta, while short, was filled with many lessons. Mother Teresa strongly encouraged me to return to the United States. So with her message in my heart, I returned to the United States.

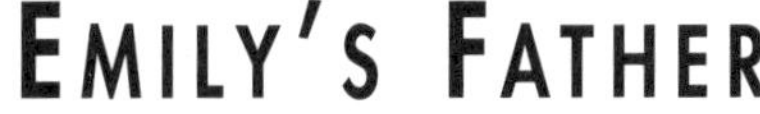

EMILY'S FATHER

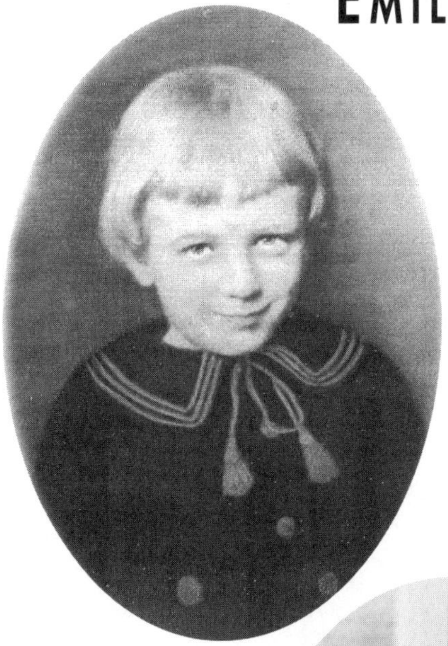

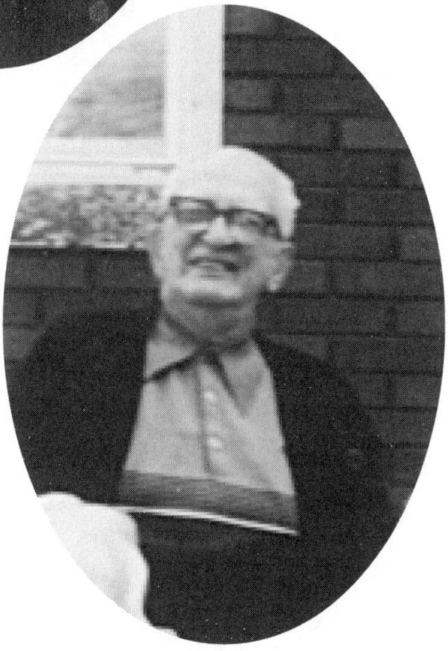

MELANCHTHEON FRANTZ ALBERT

APRIL 9, 1909 — MAY 15, 1995

My parent's marriage had not been a good one, nor had our family life been enviable. I could hardly remember anything about my father and what I could remember, I did not like. I was still haunted by Mother's last request that I forgive him. But when I thought of her life and what she had gone through, I could not. I was emotionally reminded of why I had gravitated to the field of Gerontology and the problems of our older population. Having experienced my mother's death, I found it easy to reach out to the elderly. I wanted to make a positive difference in their lives. If I can reach out to other older people, I reasoned, I should be able to reach out to my own father? I tried to think of him as just another elderly person but this strategy didn't work.

Fifteen years after Mother's death, my father found himself needing more assistance around the house. He had difficulty preparing his meals, grocery shopping, driving and maintaining his yard. He looked to his daughters for help. Veronica, my middle sister, who lived within thirty minutes of Lank, was weighed down with the demands of a full-time job as well as being a wife and a mother and thus felt she could not care for my father on a regular basis. Barbara, my oldest sister, is divorced, has four children and lived approximately 500 miles away. I lived approximately 2,200 miles from Lank and my contact with him had been limited to telephone calls and even those had been sparse since my mother died. Of the three of us, Barbara had the best relationship with our father and she was willing to take him in. But given her schedule, caring for Lank would have been extremely difficult.

Early in our marriage, George and I spoke with Lank on the telephone every two or three months. Each time, Lank would speak negatively: he never saw anyone, he was not doing well, he thought he was going to die and, on many occasions, he said he wished he were already dead. There was never a time we spoke to him that he didn't cry. As the years passed, he continued to give us the strong impression that he was a pathetic, lonely, dying old man.

While we were providing long-distance caregiving to George's father via phone and making numerous trips back to Ohio where he lived, Lank called and said he felt an urgent need to leave Pennsylvania; he didn't want to live by himself any longer. I was surprised and on edge when he said he wanted to live with one of his daughters who would care for him in his remaining years. Considering I had left home at fourteen and he had later disowned me for having interracial friends, I found it strange that he sought solace in my home. Could I provide someone who prompted so many unpleasant memories with the love and care he needed? Could I really get past the past when looking at him every day would be a reminder? I knew his move to our home would be so final for him that I had to be sure I could handle it before I said yes. But could I be sure?

After considering living with my sisters and discussing his options with them, it was clear to everyone that the lifestyle and accommodations George and I could offer would be the best for him. When Lank asked if it would be possible for him to move to Salt Lake City and live with my husband and me, I told him I could not make this decision by myself, that I would first have to speak with George. (I also needed to take a hard look at how I felt.)

When George and I discussed Lank's request, we agreed that even though he was a depressing person to speak to, there was something about him, something we can't quite explain told us we could and should help him. George reassured me we could conquer or handle anything with the love we had for each other and asked, "Wouldn't it be nice for you to share that love with Lank after all these years?" I thought to myself, what does George know? These are my emotions, my wounds and they have not healed.

I felt compelled to discuss my concerns with my priest who suggested that because of the strength he knew George and I had as a couple, we could and should open up to this challenge of love. "Remember," he said, "the power of the Holy Spirit is within each of us to handle challenges like this." Father Thomas said he would be available if I needed to talk. George reminded me that one reason we purchased our home was because it had a mother-in-law apartment in the basement and we had always said the first parent who needed or wanted to live in it could. Since Lank was the first to ask, it was OK with George if he moved in.

I had always believed if one of our parents wanted to use the basement apartment, it would be one of George's parents. In my wildest dreams had I never imagined I would reunite with my father under the same roof. But I could not refuse our home to Lank so I invited him to move to Utah. I let my father live with us, not because of my love for a parent but because of my empathy for the aged, my commitment to be a steward of life, and the emotional support I received from George. I expected to face daily challenges. Ultimately, caring for Lank gave me peace within myself and with my father.

Lank's Major Concerns

To make Lank feel at ease about the move cross country, George called him regularly to answer any and all questions he had. One major worry he had was that he would sell everything he owned, including his home, and move in with us, only to find our living arrangements would not work. "What if, after all of this, you and George decide you do not want me in your home, where would I go?" he asked me once. We told him our commitment was solid, we would always be honest with him, and if there were any differences we would all work hard to work them out. George told him this would be *his* home too and he could stay until he died; if he chose to leave, it would be entirely up to him.

Another concern was that he might not have enough money once he moved to Salt Lake City; Lank wanted to know how much we would charge him to stay with us. He told us candidly about income from Social Security and pension checks. George and I agreed we would not charge him anything. His only expenses would be gas, electricity, phone, food and incidentals. His basement apartment was wired for cable TV and he would not have to pay for hook-ups or monthly maintenance. He really felt good with these arrangements and said he was looking forward to moving out West to live with us.

Preparation Begins

When we told Lank the basement apartment was for him and he could bring with him all of his furnishings, he said he would rather bring only his clothes, pictures and television set. So George and I went to work cleaning, painting and furnishing his apartment to get it ready for his arrival. When furnishing an apartment for a parent, expenses can be held down considerably if new furniture and appliances are not a prerequisite. To furnish the apartment comfortably, we began watching for garage and used furniture sales in the classified section of the local newspaper.

It did not take long for us to find an ad placed by a well-to-do couple who had just married and were moving from their two large homes into a new, smaller one. They had a lot of beautiful furniture we were able to purchase for a fraction of what they had paid. For example, they told us they had paid

$2,100 for two end tables and a coffee table for which we paid them $150. A practically new $1,700 couch cost us $150. For their queen size bed with mattress, box springs and head board, our cost was $50. It did not take us long to furnish Lank's apartment this way and it only cost us $1,000.

Our house was now ready for Lank to move in. Everything was ready, that is, except me. Barbara had traveled to Pennsylvania to help Lank close out his home and chaperone him to Salt Lake City. Since Veronica lived close to Lank, she took responsibility for selling his home. I went to work preparing myself emotionally for his arrival. I remember thinking, "Oh God, there is nothing worse than what I am about to go through!" I was wrong because that same week I was diagnosed with breast cancer. The diagnosis sure helped me put things in perspective. It helped me see Lank's coming to live with us as a chance for us to reconcile before either of us died. Although still somewhat frightened, I was ready to work on this challenge because I needed personally to try to make something positive out of all the negative years with my father.

Exploring Surgical Options

Like many elderly people, Lank always believed what the doctor said was gospel. As a result, he didn't always make the best medical decisions for himself. Rather than act blindly, people need to get all of the facts because doctor's are not infallible. When surgery is suggested, get a second opinion. If the opinions are different, get a third opinion. Many insurance companies will encourage and pay for second and third opinions.

Just before he moved to Salt Lake City, Lank telephoned to let us know he had been diagnosed with symptomatic gallbladder disease. He was scheduled for open cholecystectomy surgery, a major operation in which the gallbladder is removed. This surgical procedure requires a ten centimeter incision under the rib cage. Recovery takes five to seven days in the hospital.

By coincidence, a couple of days before Lank's call, we had seen a commercial about laparoscopic laser cholecystectomy surgery. A local surgeon suggested laser surgery was easy on the patient, the patient would be admitted to the hospital as an outpatient and, under general endotracheal anesthesia, four small incisions would be made. The gallbladder would be removed and the patient could return home the day of the surgery or the morning after with minimal pain, wearing only an adhesive bandage over the incisions. Patients could do anything they normally would do early on with minor modification to diet. Regardless of which procedure is used, an open cholecystectomy or a laser cholecystectomy, either can lead to infection, bleeding, pulmonary problems, phlebitis, bowel injury, ductal injury and recurrent gallstones. So it made sense to have the easier surgery done.

When Lank called a second time to talk about his scheduled surgery, George called me into the living room where he was watching television. Unbelievably, the same commercial had just come on. I told Lank to hold on and had George write down the doctor's phone number so we could call later. We told Lank about the commercial and how easy it made the operation sound. We suggested he call his Pennsylvania doctor and cancel his surgery, at least until we were able to check out this local doctor and his new procedure. Lank said he would make the call first thing in the morning.

While Lank spoke with his doctor in Pennsylvania we were talking with the doctor in Salt Lake City. He assured us the new procedure would be, by far, much easier than the open cholecystectomy on someone Lank's age. I telephoned Lank and suggested he come to Salt Lake City for a consultation with the doctor, and he should plan to stay and not return to Pennsylvania. Lank liked our suggestion, so I contacted my sisters and told them we were moving up our plans to relocate our father out West.

When Lank arrived in Salt Lake City he was moved to tears when we showed him his new home. The first thing we did, after we got him settled into his apartment was make an appointment for him to see the doctor. When they met we discovered that, just as we had expected, Lank was an excellent candidate for the laparoscopic cholecystectomy procedure. The doctor scheduled the surgery and, true to his words, Lank was in and out of the hospital the same day his gallbladder was removed. Lank left the hospital wearing a Band-Aid about the size of a dime over each of the four tiny stitched incisions. He never had any discomfort and was able to eat, drink and move about freely right away.

Sometimes people are fearful to research alternatives to medical problems. They may have difficulties understanding the differences in their options or pride may keep them from inquiring fully. You can assist someone by aiding in research and taking time to clearly explain procedures and treatments in detail. As a friend they may feel more comfortable in asking you questions rather than asking the doctor.

LANK'S MEDICAL HISTORY

Once Lank moved in with us, we realized he had many long-term health problems he had never tried to do anything about. Lank started smoking when he was eight and he said he would never give it up. He always complained of leg pain. On occasion the doctor would explain to him that the nicotine in his cigarettes acted as a vasoconstrictor, restricting the flow of blood to the lower part of his legs, thus contributing to his pain. Regardless of what the doctor said, no degree of discomfort could discourage Lank from smoking. By his late sixties, he had developed peripheral vascular disease necessitating a femoral bypass to the arteries of both legs. Between the femoral bypasses and smoking, his circulation never returned to normal.

At an early age Lank had perforated an ear drum which was never corrected. He also had all his teeth removed as a young man. He wore only upper dentures in his later years because his lower plate had been inadvertently flushed down the toilet and he refused to pay to have it replaced. He took medication for hypertension and suffered from numerous bone spurs on the bottom of his feet. Tired of the daily trouble of putting in and taking out contact lenses, he chose to wear very thick corrective eyeglasses.

Of all Lank's physical problems, his feet gave him his biggest discomfort. The doctor found three things wrong with Lank's feet. First, Lank had four or five pointed bone spurs in the heal of each foot. They looked like thumb tacks sticking into the fleshy part of his heal, and without question they were part of the reason Lank's feet hurt. But removing the spurs required surgery; he chose not to have them removed. Lank's doctor suggested orthotics as an alternative to help ease his foot pain. These shoe inserts were constructed from a plastic mold of Lank's feet, and would help distribute his weight so that the bone spurs would not press into the fleshy part of his heal. Lank chose the orthotics over surgery and they did alleviate some of his foot pain.

The second thing the doctor found was Lank had broken down arches, probably from wearing shoes that were too large. Over a number of years, he had a pinched nerve that ran between his big toe and his second toe and a shot of cortisone was the only thing the doctor could recommend for treatment. Lank agreed to try the cortisone, but while it decreased the pain, his discomfort never went away entirely.

Lank had the insurance and the money to replace his dental plate, purchase a hearing aid, buy new glasses and do something to reduce the pain of his bone spurs, but he elected to do nothing. Either he did not want to spend the money on himself or he did not want to impose by asking another person to take him to the doctor. It also is possible he did not know how to find an appropriate doctor or was afraid the doctor would tell him he needed surgery.

Lank always blindly followed the recommendations of doctors. Even though he knew he did not want surgery, Lank thought that if the doctor suggested it he would be "forced" to go through with it. When I asked him why he never took better care of his body, Lank just shrugged it off—it was not important to him.

As soon as it became evident there was a medical problem developing, we would let Lank know we would help him explore his available options. Then, we would immediately contact his physician (or nurse) so they could attend to his needs. Chances are that when Lank was not feeling well, he would do nothing.

Even though Lank did very little to help himself, it was his right to be a part of the decision-making process and to determine what course of action would be taken, if any. After all, it was his body. As far as we could see, he never stopped complaining about the things that caused him problems, but not willing to change the personal habits that contributed to his aches and pains, always relied on someone else to solve things.

Lank's attitude toward taking care of himself is not unusual for his generation: for people who survived raising a family during the Depression, saving money was a priority. These folks are more likely, when cost is involved, to consider only what they cannot live without, not what would make their lives more pleasurable.

Commitments and Routines

Never make a commitment to your parents lightly because you can be sure they won't take commitments lightly. With elderly parents you soon realize that what may not seem important to you is a major issue for them, especially parents dependent on you for transportation and social interaction. Your parents will cling to every commitment you make. So your commitments have to fit your schedule as well as accommodate your parents' limitations.

While George and I were juggling timetables, trying to work full-time, we were tending two homes and trying to meet the varying needs of three parents (at this time we were still providing long-distance care for George's father in Ohio, helping George's mother so she could continue to maintain her Salt Lake home and caring for Lank in our home). In all this, each of our parents was looking only at their individual timeframes. When we told Lank we would do something for him, he took that as a total commitment. He always reminded us of what we were going to do for him and then pinned us down to a time. The adjustment for Lank, as for all our parents, was having to live on someone else's schedule. The adjustment for us was having three people reminding us almost daily of what we committed to do for them.

We solved our main time problem by recognizing our parent's limitations and utilizing that knowledge in a logical and practical way. For example, since they moved slowly, we prepared early, but let them get around on their own. If they were confused, we helped them get ready and used a wheelchair. If incontinence was a problem, we checked with them frequently and took them to the toilet often.

Like commitments, routines are an important part of life. Even though our parents had to learn to live on our schedule, they were still able to maintain some control of their lives by keeping to their routines. Everyone has a routine, even though he or she may not be aware of it. For example, my father had a number of routines he followed, day and night. These routines helped give order to his life. Every Tuesday Lank had two eggs, four strips of bacon, one cup of coffee and a slice of toast for breakfast. He never changed this menu. Likewise, other daily meals were regular and the same each week. Even though he occasionally missed a particular meal, Lank would not deviate from the eating routine for the rest of the day. Lank had two candy kisses at 10 a.m., never more, never less. He ate dinner at 4 p.m. He walked two blocks each day, always towards the west, never the east. He rode his stationery bike ten miles a day, never more, never less. Every day from 6 to 7 p.m., he watched *Wheel of Fortune* and *Jeopardy*, no matter who was visiting him. He went to bed at 9 p.m. tired or not and, if he couldn't sleep, he took something to help.

Humans are creatures of habit. Routines are normal and healthy and are needed to maintain some sense of order in our lives. Routines develop confidence in the elderly just as they do in children. They may thus be important coping strategies for the elderly. If a behavior is inappropriate, if habits are annoying or create a health problem, like spitting into various objects throughout the house, or digging out impactions, then discuss the problem with your parent. Otherwise, be sensitive and understanding.

George in the Insurance Maze

At the very least, insurance can be difficult to understand and it is easy to get so caught up in the frustrating, time consuming maze of procedures and requirements that you lose sight of the issue: having adequate insurance. It is important to know what insurance coverage parents have and if their insurance policies will be beneficial to them in case they need hospitalization or nursing home care. Aside from Medicare, a secondary or supplemental insurance policy is extremely important, so long as it provides needed additional coverage. Be aware that more is not always better. Medicare generally pays eighty percent of medical bills. Additional policies should pay the twenty percent of charges Medicare does not cover. This is referred to as filling the Medicare Gap. If the elderly do not have enough coverage to fill this gap, they do not have enough insurance.

We were told about an elderly woman who purchased six insurance policies from one company. When she fell and broke her neck, not one of those policies covered her injury. When choosing supplemental insurance, quality, not quantity is the issue: one excellent secondary or supplemental insurance policy is all that is necessary. Make sure your parents have one and make sure you know what it will and will not cover. Contact a number of insurance companies and compare plans. If you are not clear about plan differences, get in touch with someone who can help you get what you want and need. That someone can be a professional person, a relative or a friend. George's experience with the insurance companies will show you how complex the "insurance maze" can be.

Although it can be dangerous to have too little insurance, it is also easy to end up paying for more insurance than one really needs. Lank had too much coverage, and because George was not only processing his insurance, but also insurance matters for his parents and for me, it took him quite some time to realize Lank's insurance could be reduced as well as streamlined. George was "lost in the maze" of Lank's insurance. We hope his experience, and the lessons he learned, will help you save time, energy and frustration.

Some providers of services do not bill secondary or supplemental insurance companies directly. For those who do, the responsibility for paying that bill and following up on the insurance payment remains with the patient until it is paid. This was the case with Lank. So when the medical statements and the *Explanation of Your Medicare Benefits* (EOMB) notices started coming to our home after Lank's cholecystectomy, he asked George to help him with the insurance forms because he didn't understand them.

After discussing his insurance problems, George told Lank not to worry because he would process all the insurance papers for him. George knew Lank was on Medicare, but didn't know if he kept secondary insurance with his retirement package or if he had purchased a supplemental insurance; either policy would pay what Medicare didn't. Lank said when he retired he kept an excellent secondary insurance policy with Metropolitan Life. He also had a supplemental insurance policy with Blue Cross/Blue Shield of Pennsylvania which he had been carrying since his retirement nineteen years earlier.

Here's how George got lost. When he filled out Lank's insurance forms initially, he didn't take into account that one policy was secondary and the other supplemental. On the Metropolitan form, George answered yes when asked if the patient was covered by another group benefit plan. When asked for the name of the other insurance company, he typed in the name, Pennsylvania address and policy number of Lank's supplemental policy insurer, Blue Cross. On the Blue Cross form when asked if the patient was covered by another group plan, he again responded yes and dutifully typed in Metropolitan, Lank's secondary policyholder, the Metropolitan policy number and the company address. Without knowing it at the time, by crosslisting policies on different forms, George was creating what would be a frustrating and confusing situation for himself as well as for the insurance company employees.

A few days later George took another wrong turn in the insurance maze. Lank asked if they could discuss his medical insurance. He needed to renew his insurance with Blue Cross. George told him he would call the Blue Cross office in Salt Lake City to see what he had to do and how much it would cost to get it renewed. That was the easy part. George had no problem contacting a Blue Cross representative in Utah. The representative said she would send an application and, sure enough, a few days later the form arrived. George filled it out and had Lank sign it, enclosed Lank's $80 payment for the first month and mailed the completed application. Lank's Blue Cross of Utah policy arrived a week later at about the same time the one in Pennsylvania expired.

George assumed that because Blue Cross is a national company, moving from one state to another would not mean a change in the policy number or payment process. He was wrong and this misunderstanding eventually led to the realization Lank really did not need his Blue Cross policy.

From the very beginning we had problems with Blue Cross of Pennsylvania. We were confused. The people at Metropolitan and Blue Cross were confused. Everyone was confused. To start with, Blue Cross did not pay their portion of the bills, or at least that's what we thought. When George contacted the Blue Cross office in Salt Lake City he was told to contact the Blue Cross office in Pennsylvania because that was where Lank's bills were handled. He did not realize then that they were referring him to Pennsylvania for payment only because Lank's Blue Cross Pennsylvania address and policy number were on the original set of insurance forms George had sent them. He thought the people at Blue Cross in Salt Lake City were telling him they had a national billing office in Pennsylvania.

Actually, each state has its own Blue Cross program. For example, if you live in Utah, you buy your policy in Utah and have your paperwork processed in Salt Lake City. From an administrative point-of-view, Blue Cross operates on a franchise system. Because George had filled out and made extra copies of Lank's Pennsylvania Blue Cross forms, he was inadvertently using Lank's Pennsylvania policy number and address when submitting claims to Blue Cross of Utah.

There's another confusing point. As long as Lank's Pennsylvania policy was in effect, George should have been sending his statements directly to Pennsylvania rather than to the Salt Lake City office, even though he was receiving medical services in Salt Lake City. Once Lank obtained a policy with Blue Cross of Utah and his Pennsylvania policy was no longer valid, his claims then should have been submitted to the Salt Lake City office with his Salt Lake City policy number on them.

Furthermore, Blue Cross did not need to pay first on any of Lank's claims: his secondary insurance was with Metropolitan. Blue Cross knew Metropolitan would pay whatever Medicare didn't. And, as a supplemental insurance, Blue Cross had little, if any, responsibility for paying any claim before Metropolitan. Blue Cross would be responsible only if Metropolitan did not fully pay the twenty percent Medicare doesn't cover. The likelihood of this happening is very slim.

During this period, when George had all three of Lank's insurance policy identification cards in front of him, and after hours of long-distance phone calls and hours spent writing letters to Blue Cross of Pennsylvania, a huge light bulb suddenly flashed inside his head. If Lank had a secondary insurance policy with Metropolitan, why then was he carrying a supplemental insurance policy with Blue Cross? To find out why, George called Blue Cross of Utah and asked their representative this question directly. His suspicion was confirmed. She said Lank did not need the supplemental coverage.

We found out Lank's insurance policy with Blue Cross had rarely been used because service providers sent his secondary insurance to Metropolitan, which paid after the primary carrier, Medicare. Lank had been paying into Blue Cross of Pennsylvania for nineteen years and he had never been told by any agent he did not need the policy (granted Lank probably never asked and Blue Cross may not have known another policy existed). Lank had paid approximately $80 a month for a supplemental insurance policy that did him no good, and there was no way he could recover that loss. In any kind of a savings program, what Lank paid in premiums over a nineteen year period would have made a pretty respectable savings account by today's standards.

George got lost wandering in the "insurance maze." We are certain Lank would have given up in frustration long before he realized his coverage with Blue Cross was worthless to him. And he would have continued to pay $80 a month for a policy he did not need.

Special Power of Attorney and Living Wills

The Special Power of Attorney and the Living Will are probably the least understood documents for the elderly and their caregivers. The following explanation is provided, in part, with information gathered from Utah Legal Services, Inc., Utah Area Agencies on Aging, Utah Medical Association Foundation, and the Utah Health Care Association.

The Living Will is a legal document that expresses the wishes of the person signing the document, called the declarant. It indicates the declarant does not want life artificially prolonged by life-sustaining procedures. The will is certified by two physicians who must personally examine the declarant, and determine that the application of life-sustaining procedures would serve only to unnaturally prolong the moment of death and unnaturally postpone or prolong the dying process.

A life-sustaining procedure, as defined by law, means any medical procedure or intervention which, in the judgment of the attending physician, serves only to prolong the dying process when applied to a person who has a terminal condition. Under a Living Will, any time the declarant has an injury, disease or illness, which is certified in writing to be a terminal condition or persistent vegetative state, the declarant directs that these procedures be withheld or withdrawn and his or her death be permitted to occur naturally. The Living Will is of no use without two physician's stating in the medical records that the patient is suffering a terminal condition. Without such a signed statement, paramedics responding to an emergency call will do CPR or any other procedures they deem necessary to save the person's life. When the patient arrives at the hospital, the attending physician may then confirm the patient is in a terminal condition. If so, he or she will then ask a second physician to confirm the diagnosis and life support systems will be discontinued.

The Special Power of Attorney, which we obtained from three of our parents, includes a specific medical treatment plan and gave us general permission to make medical decisions on our parent's behalf. It is less limiting than the Living Will, and it is more effective in preventing CPR or any other heroics or life-sustaining procedures being done against the declarant's wishes. The Special Power of Attorney appoints another person as an agent for all medical treatment decisions, not just treatment of a terminal illness, when the declarant is unable to communicate. It is our opinion that the Special Power of Attorney is the preferable document if it is the declarant's intention not to have heroics performed in the case of any life threatening injury, disease or illness. The medical treatment plan included within the Special Power of Attorney is a legally binding directive to physicians and providers of medical services that describes what medical care and treatment is to be provided or withheld.

Medical treatment directives can be simple statements like:

> In the event of a sudden life threatening emergency, do not resuscitate (DNR). No Code. No Heroics. Do not use respirators, ventilators or administer medication other than those medications necessary to prevent infection, provide comfort or alleviate pain.

When an elderly person does not want medical personnel to perform life-sustaining procedures, having the Special Power of Attorney and Medical Treatment Plan available allows the paramedics to concentrate on keeping the patient comfortable while transporting him or her to the hospital. Once at the hospital, the physician must respect the patient's wishes and honor the Special Power of Attorney.

To validate the Special Power of Attorney, it only needs to be notarized by a notary public. To validate the medical treatment plan, which is a part of the Special Power of Attorney, the document must have been signed in the presence of two adult witnesses and signed by the attending physician. Witnesses may not be related to the declarant by blood or marriage, or entitled to any part of the declarant's estate. Witnesses may not be directly financially responsible for the declarant's medical care, nor agents of any health care facility in which the declarant is cared for at the time of signing. The original medical treatment plan should be given to the declarant's physician and a copy should be provided to the person the declarant has empowered with his or her Special Power of Attorney.

Sample documents—a Special Power of Attorney, Medical Treatment Plan and Living Will available through the state Medical Association—are included on the following pages. Remember, this is an overview of the Living Will and the Special Power of Attorney. Keep in mind that the laws may vary widely from state to state. To investigate the situation in your own state, consider consulting legal counsel.

SPECIAL POWER OF ATTORNEY

Appointment of an agent for all medical treatment decisions (*not* just in case of a terminal illness) when I am unable to speak for myself.

I, ____, residing at

____,

on this _____ day of _______________, 19____, being of sound mind, willfully and voluntarily appoint ______________________________,

residing at ____,

as my agent and attorney-in-fact, without substitution, with lawful authority to execute a Medical Treatment Plan on my behalf pursuant to Utah Code Ann. 75-2-1105, governing the care and treatment to be administered to or withheld from me at any time after I incur an injury, disease or illness which renders me unable to give current medical directions to attending physicians and other providers of medical services.

I have carefully selected this agent with confidence in the belief that this person's familiarity with my desires, beliefs and attitudes will result in directions to attending physicians and providers of health care which would probably be the same as I would give, were I able to do so.

This power of attorney shall become effective and remain in effect from the time my attending physician certifies that I have incurred a physical or mental condition rendering me unable to give current directions to attending physicians and other providers of health care as to my care and treatment.

____
Principal's signature

____
Address

____
City/State

— continued —

Special Power of Attorney
Page 2

STATE OF UTAH)
:SS.
COUNTY OF_____________________________)

On the __________day of ___________________, 19____, personally appeared before me ____ who proved to me his/her identity through documentary evidence in the form of ____ to be the person whose name is signed on the foregoing power of attorney, and who duly acknowledged to me that he/she has read and fully understands the foregoing power of attorney, executed the same of his/her own volition and for the purposes set forth, and that he/she was acting under no constraint or undue influence whatsoever.

____
NOTARY PUBLIC
STATE OF UTAH

My Commission expires:

Date: _____/_____/___________

(Pursuant to Utah Code Ann. 75-2-1106)

MEDICAL TREATMENT PLAN

I, ____, certify that I am the attending physician for ______________________________________ of ______________________________________, who is presently under my care this ______ day of ________________, 19___ and who has been under my care since the ________ day of ________________, 19___.

The declarant, the above-named patient, is currently suffering from the following injury, disease or illness: ______________________________

____

____

I certify that I have explained to the declarant, to the extent he/she is able to understand, and to the available person(s) acting as proxy, the reasonably available alternatives for care and treatment. I certify that the care and treatment alternatives directed below are:

_____ directed by the declarant; or

_____ that the declarant has a physical or mental condition which renders him/her unable to give personal directions for care and treatment and that the care and treatment alternatives directed below are, in my opinion and in the opinion of the declarant's proxy, what the declarant would probably decide if able to give current directions concerning his/her care and treatment.

Date: _____/_____/_______ __________________________________

Signature of Attending Physician

The following care and treatment or withholding of treatment is directed with respect to the declarant: ____________________________

____

____

____

Relationship to declarant of any agent signing for declarant, if applicable	Signature of declarant or authorized agent

____

____

____

Address of signer, including city, county and state of residence

— continued —

Medical Treatment Plan
Page 2

We, the witnesses, certify that each of us is 18 years of age or older; that we personally witnessed the declarant or a proxy sign this directive; that we are acquainted with the declarant and believe that care and treatment alternatives directed above are what the declarant has decided for himself/herself concerning his/her care and treatment, or, if the foregoing was signed by a proxy, that we are acquainted with the proxy and believe that the proxy sincerely believes that the care and treatment alternatives directed above are what the declarant would probably decide for himself/herself if able to give current directions concerning his/her care and treatment; that neither of us signed the above directive for or on behalf of declarant; that we are not related to the declarant by blood or marriage nor are we entitled to any portion of declarant's estate according to the laws of intestate succession of this state or under any Will or Codicil of the declarant; that we are not agents of any health care facility in which declarant may be a patient at the time of signing this directive; and that we are not directly financially responsible for declarant's medical care.

Witness #1	**Witness #2**
Signature	Signature
Name (please print)	Name (please print)
Address	Address
City/State/Zip Code	City/State/Zip Code

(Pursuant to Utah Code Ann. 75-2-1105)

LIVING WILL

1. On this ________ day of ___________________________, 19______, I, ___________________________, being of sound mind, hereby willfully and voluntarily make known my desire that my life not be artificially prolonged by life-sustaining procedures except as I may otherwise provide in this directive. I understand that the term "life-sustaining procedure," as defined by law, i) means any medical procedure or intervention which, when applied to a person who has a terminal condition would, in the judgment of the attending physician, serve only to prolong the dying process, ii) does not mean medication, sustenance, or medical procedures for providing comfort care or for alleviating pain, unless I so specify below.

2. I declare that if at any time I should have an injury, disease or illness, which is certified in writing to be a terminal condition or persistent vegetative state by two physicians who have personally examined me, and in the opinion of those physicians the application of life-sustaining procedures would serve only to unnaturally prolong the moment of my death and to unnaturally postpone or prolong the dying process, I direct that these procedures be withheld or withdrawn and my death be permitted to occur naturally.

3. I expressly intend this directive to be a final expression of my legal right to refuse medical or surgical treatment and to accept the consequences from this refusal, which shall remain in effect notwithstanding my future inability to give current medical directions to treating physicians and other providers of medical services.

4. I understand that the term "life-sustaining procedure" includes artificial nutrition and hydration and any other procedures that I specify below to be considered life-sustaining but does not include the administration of medication or the performance of any medical procedure which is intended to provide comfort care or to alleviate pain: ______

____

____

5. I reserve the right to give current medical directions to physicians and other providers of medical services so long as I am able, even though these directions may conflict with the above-written directive that life-sustaining procedures be withheld or withdrawn.

6. I understand the full import of this directive and declare that I am emotionally and mentally competent to make this directive.

____

Declarant Signature

____

City/County/State of Residence

— continued —

Living Will
Page 2

We, the witnesses, certify that each of us is 18 years of age or older and each personally witnessed the declarant sign or direct the signing of this directive; that we are acquainted with the declarant and believe him/her to be of sound mind; that the declarant's desires are as expressed above; that neither of us is a person who signed the above directive on behalf of the declarant; that we are not related to the declarant by blood or marriage nor are we entitled to any portion of declarant's estate according to the laws of intestate succession of this state or under any Will or Codicil of the declarant; that we are not directly financially responsible for declarant's medical care; and that we are not agents of any health care facility in which the declarant may be a patient at the time of signing this directive.

Witness #1	**Witness #2**
______________________	______________________
Signature	Signature
______________________	______________________
Name (please print)	Name (please print)
______________________	______________________
Address	Address
______________________	______________________
City/State/Zip Code	City/State/Zip Code

(Pursuant to Utah Code Ann. 75-2-1104)

The Obvious is not so Obvious: Changes in Behavior as Signals

When caring for the elderly, expect the unexpected and don't take anything for granted because what appears to be the obvious will sometimes turn out not to be. Let me explain. Caregivers may be unaware that a parent, in their presence, is experiencing a heart attack, stroke or other serious problems. This happened with George and I when Lank had his stroke. Initially, we were caught off guard: we thought he was either in a bad mood or upset with us. In just a short time, however, we realized there was something wrong.

George and I had just arrived home and George went downstairs to check on Lank. When George knocked on the apartment door, Lank did not respond with his usual "come in," so George opened the door and asked if anyone was home. This time, Lank answered, "Yeah." As George entered the living room, he felt certain there was something wrong because Lank's voice and mannerisms were different from anything George could remember. George asked Lank simple questions like, "How was your day? What did you have for breakfast? How do you feel?" He did not like Lank's answers or demeanor. It seemed to George there was something wrong. He called me to come downstairs.

George waited to see how Lank would respond to my questions. As I entered Lank's apartment, I hollered out as I normally did, "Helloooo." I knew immediately something was wrong because he would always answer with the same, "Helloooo." This time, he did not respond at all. I asked questions similar to those George had already asked and I received the same kinds of answers. I too was convinced something was wrong. We tried to get Lank to stand and walk, but he was unable to rise. It was only then that we thought either Lank had had a stroke or he was in the process of having one. George called 911.

We told Lank an ambulance would arrive shortly to take him to the hospital because we thought he might be having or may have had a stroke. We were taken totally by surprise when all of a sudden Lank stood up and walked to the bathroom, when only moments before he could not even stand. George and I looked at each other in shock. Lank was gone for about three minutes and as he returned an ambulance and a fire engine were pulling up in front of our home with their sirens wailing. Lank was sitting in his lift chair when the paramedics entered his apartment. We explained what we observed in Lank's answers and mannerisms. Then the paramedics asked Lank what we took for granted he would not be able to answer, but he easily answered. Questions like, "What is your name? How are you feeling? What day is it? What did you have for breakfast?" George and I could not believe what we were hearing. We certainly didn't expect to hear the answers Lank was giving. We told the paramedics we could not give any explanation for why there was this sudden change in him. The change back to coherence was definitely unexpected.

The paramedics could find nothing wrong with Lank but they were required to take him to the hospital for observation and to confirm there was nothing wrong. George and I followed the ambulance to the hospital. The emergency room doctor couldn't find anything wrong and had no idea what had happened. He said we could take Lank home. The paramedics advised us that if a similar episode occurred again, we should wait for about an hour and, if there was no change, call and have Lank returned to the hospital.

While the three of us were in Lank's apartment discussing the situation we had just experienced, Lank lit a cigarette, took one drag, then let it slip from his fingers to the floor. This time Lank was totally unaware of where he was or what was happening. We recalled what the paramedics had told us: if a similar situation should occur, wait one hour. Approximately five minutes had elapsed when George said, "Emily, if we don't do something now, Lank may not be alive in an hour. There is no question; he needs help." Because we felt sure this time that Lank was experiencing a stroke, I agreed. So once again, we called 911 and Lank was rushed to the hospital.

While being admitted to the hospital, Lank's physician ordered a series of tests to determine the extent of Lank's problem. The results showed Lank had experienced three or four mini-strokes but presently he was not in a life-or-death situation. Still, he needed to stay in the hospital for a few days. During his hospital stay, Lank had an occupational and physical therapist working with him ninety minutes daily. Because there was not as much damage done as was first thought and because of the therapist's efforts and the care the hospital was giving him, Lank showed continuous improvement and was soon to be released.

After a stay of only eight days, Lank returned home where both a physical and an occupational therapist continued treating Lank to help him regain his strength and range of motion. In addition to the therapist, an aide assisted Lank three times a week with bathing, cleaning his bathroom and making his bed. The aide also prepared one meal a day and cleaned up after Lank was finished eating.

To make Lank's apartment safer during his recovery, scatter rugs were removed, telephone wires secured and grab bars installed in the bathroom. Determined to regain his strength, Lank returned to his daily walks outdoors. But against the therapist's orders, Lank insisted on walking outside without a companion and he continually tripped and fell in very familiar areas. While the therapy helped him cognitively, he fought other frustrations as well such as not being able to shave himself. Because of his difficulty in handling eating utensils and opening some containers, eating became a chore for him. Although there are devices available to help stroke victims with eating and opening containers, Lank struggled without using these devices because for him the devices were not tools but degrading reminders of what he could not do. Over the next few months, as he tried to regain what he had lost both physically and mentally, his struggles and challenges continued.

George and I had some hands-on experience working with stroke victims. As students in the University of Utah Gerontology Program, we were required to do a practicum. Our practicum required we each spend 200 hours working with the elderly in an agency or facility of our choice. This allowed us a practical hands-on approach to learning about caring for various health problems of the aged. We chose the Professional Rehabilitation Center (PRC) to do the first 100 hours. Using the knowledge we gained at PRC on how to care for a stroke victim, we were able to assist Lank every day with his therapy.

After experiencing Lank's stroke episode, we learned never to take anything for granted. We continually observed our parents, knowing that differences in their behavior could be signals of serious health problems or emergencies. And we constantly remind ourselves the signs are not always obvious.

Choices: Emergency Medical Service Personnel or Home Health Services

When a medical emergency arises and you call 911 for assistance, be prepared for the emergency medical technician (EMT) who responds to the call to do cardiopulmonary resuscitation (CPR), or other necessary heroics, to save the life of your parent. If a person's heart were to stop a paramedic would be legally obligated to use everything within his or her power to see that the person lived until safely delivered to the hospital. For those who do not want any heroics, it is important to have a Special Power of Attorney Medical Treatment plan displayed in a conspicuous place, such as on the wall above the head of the bed. EMTs' first obligation is to save lives; they won't wait while others search for a medical treatment document. However, do not assume that just because you have a document displayed, it will be honored. We found some EMTs do not know or misunderstand what documents to honor when responding to an emergency call.

Some states have made it easier for 911 EMT's to identify a patient's right to self-determination when a physician previously has determined a person to be terminally ill. For example, the Utah state legislature passed and implemented an extension to the Living Will Act in May 1993. The purpose of the legislation is to give pre-hospital personnel a simple and easy way to recognize a patient's right to self-determination concerning CPR and other emergency care procedures. The law was sponsored by the American College of Emergency Physicians and submitted to the legislature by the Bureau of Emergency Medical Services, Utah Department of Health. It established the Emergency Medical Services Do Not Resuscitate (EMS/DNR) program which applies to cardiac and/or respiratory arrest in the patient as it relates to a *terminal* condition previously determined by a physician. If the patient meets the criteria and does not want any heroics, his or her physician will provide documentation with a bracelet or necklace identifying the patient as an EMS/DNR declarant.

The Bureau of Emergency Medical Service Staff made many efforts to educate professionals about the EMS/DNR program. Information was placed in the Utah Medical Association (UMA) newsletter and all three major Utah television stations carried segments regarding the program. Numerous conferences and workshops have been sponsored to educate individuals who provide home health care and hospice care because these people care for terminal patients. Pamphlets explaining the EMS/DNR program were left with them as well. However, requests to address the Utah Medical

Association convention and to have a display booth at the convention were politely denied.

We found not all EMT and other healthcare professionals know how the EMS/DNR program works. However, EMTs in Utah have been trained to seek Special Power of Attorney documents and with proof of status, should honor these documents. So check with the state health department to determine what medical treatment plans are acceptable in the state where your parents live.

An elderly couple confronted with a life or death situation will probably act instinctively and call 911 for help even if they do not want heroics. Our next door neighbors were an elderly couple; the women was in her seventies, the man in his eighties. The husband had a heart attack in his living room while his wife was present. She called 911. My neighbor's wife insisted she only wanted to keep her husband free from pain.

Through the windows I watched as the paramedics and firemen rushed into the house. They exited just as quickly with my neighbor's body on a stretcher. The paramedics worked hard to revive my friend. While it seemed like a lifetime, I'm sure it was only a matter of minutes as I watched one paramedic pump the man's chest while the other administered oxygen. They prepared pads to administer electric shock in hopes of starting his heart. They zapped him a couple of times, then drove off in the ambulance.

I hurried next door so his wife would not be alone until family members arrived. She told me her husband was dead when he was removed from the house (and before the paramedics began trying to revive him). Her daughter later confirmed this story.

Watching this series of events and seeing how traumatic it was for his wife to witness them reinforced my belief that we need to educate our parents of the importance of the Special Power of Attorney. The medical treatment plan needs to be kept in a conspicuous place if it is to protect them from the emotional, confusing situation our neighbor experienced.

Both the EMS/DNR document with bracelet/necklace and the Special Power of Attorney Medical Treatment plan should be honored by EMTs, but take nothing for granted. Investigate what programs and documents are required in your state. It is our understanding that as of July 1996, the Emergency Medical Service/ Do Not Resuscitate program is used in the following states: Alaska, Arizona, Arkansas, California, Florida, Georgia, Hawaii, Idaho, Illinois, Kansas, Maine, Maryland, Missouri, Montana, New Mexico, New York, North Carolina, South Carolina, Tennessee, Utah, Washington, West Virginia and Wyoming. Remember, the EMS/DNR directive only applies to cardiac or respiratory arrest as it relates to the patient's terminal condition. For anyone not diagnosed with terminal illnesses, yet still not wanting heroics, consider a Special Power of Attorney Medical Treatment plan.

When the goal is to provide comfort to a dying person who is not diagnosed with a terminal illness, there may be better options than calling emergency medical services personnel. You can call your home health nurse who can set up IV solutions, administer antibiotics and pain killers and honor your parent's wishes as outlined. However, you must still have the Special Power of Attorney visible. When home health staff respond to oversee major procedures such as IV medication or when catheter replacement is needed, Medicare will cover 100 percent of the costs whereas Medicare pays eighty percent and you pay twenty percent of hospital costs.

The physician is the key to ensuring a person's wishes are carried out. If someone you care for does not want heroics, explore with his or her doctor the possibility of having pain control medication available in the event of an emergency. Contact your home health agency and have a nurse sent to your home to evaluate the seriousness of the situation. The nurse can report his or her findings to the doctor who can issue orders for medication at home to provide comfort care and to alleviate pain. If you are not utilizing a home health service, call your physician to make arrangements for a nurse to evaluate your parent.

Smoking After a Stroke

Don't expect lifelong smokers to quit cold turkey. People who smoke have a difficult time quitting and the longer they have smoked the more difficult it is. If you want to experience strained relations and add stress to your household, just issue commands about quitting or where smoking is allowed. You will be met with strong resistance when you set new smoking boundaries with parents who have smoked for years. So be flexible when finding solutions to control smoking in your home and, to maintain harmony, involve everyone in the decision-making process.

When Lank came to Salt Lake City to live, we knew how important smoking was to him. Over seventy-five years, starting at age eight, he had smoked one to two packs of cigarettes per day. Now that he only smoked six cigarettes a day, he wasn't about to give up the one thing he enjoyed. Nevertheless, we told him we would feel more comfortable if he would not smoke in the house when he was alone. We told him we were worried that if he was smoking alone and had another stroke, he might start a fire.

Lank was visibly upset with our suggestion, he responded by saying he wasn't concerned about a fire, and didn't care if he burned to death. I reacted, "Thank You Very Much, but you are not the only one living in this house. You may not care about yourself, but George and I care. Besides, neither of us want to die by fire." I suggested he wait until someone was with him to smoke or if he couldn't wait, go outside. In a joking way, he said it was too hot in the summer and too cold in the winter to smoke outside. Suddenly, he became very serious. He told us he should have stayed in Pennsylvania where he could have smoked anywhere and anytime he wanted. I asked him if he was serious and in anger and frustration, he answered, "Yes!" I acknowledged it must be difficult to be in the position he was in, but I didn't think smoking outside or waiting until someone was with him was asking a lot.

I reminded Lank that he only smoked six cigarettes a day and only took six drags from each cigarette, that he could dress warmly and his time outside would be minimal. If he continued to progress with his therapy, and his physical abilities returned as they were before his stroke, he could return to smoking in his apartment. His reaction to us was negative at first, but because we both expressed our feelings, discussed the problem of smoking and set a goal for him, Lank agreed to do as we asked. Imagine what it would have been like if we had excluded him from the discussion and taken his cigarettes away.

In search of an alternative to smoking outside, George suggested we call the fire department to see if they could suggest a fire-retardant that would make it safer for Lank to smoke inside by treating his living room chair and carpet. The Fire Marshall recommended a local paint store where we purchased two containers of a retardant and applied two applications: soaking Lank's lift chair and carpet, then allowing twenty-four hours to dry. Lank could now smoke safely in his apartment because any burning ashes falling on the chair or carpet would extinguish without starting a fire. If ashes fell in his lap, hopefully, he would be alert enough to put them out before he was burned: we realized there would be no guarantee. As an added safeguard, we placed a smoke alarm on the living room wall. We made a commitment to him when we told him if he recovered his health he could smoke whenever he wanted and we kept it. Over the next few weeks, Lank recovered significantly and was pretty much his old self. We gave him the go-ahead to smoke and smoke where he felt most comfortable—in his living room—watching television.

Earlier, I had explained our smoking dilemma to a priest and a university professor and both suggested we do essentially the same thing: tell our father that he did as we said or we would place him in a nursing home—something we believed to be an inappropriate solution to the problem. Threats and intimidation seldom work; they only create a hostile environment or fears.

When a dangerous situation is possible, you need to negotiate for an appropriate solution by understanding both sides of the problem. Share your concerns but also be patient and try to understand what you are asking your parent to give up. Always look for a solution by reviewing all the options and choosing the one that is best for all concerned. This process is paramount for maintaining safety *and* trust levels.

When a Walk Becomes a Shuffle: Avoiding Falls

It is dangerous for frail elderly people to walk unassisted because it takes great concentration for them just to stand; walking requires even more effort. When walking, many seniors have difficulty lifting their feet while moving forward. They slide, rather than lift and step out. Sliding gives a false sense of confidence and is a major reason obstacles such as throw rugs, telephone wires, electrical cords and so on should be removed from the floor. Broken concentration and quick changes of direction while walking forward cause most falls. Tripping over objects is another major cause.

To help those you care for maintain as much independence as they can for as long as they can, it is important to help them maintain mobility. Positioning furniture to assist them in moving about their home is one way. Chairs can be used for balancing or for resting. Know your parents' limitations and be creative.

One evening George and I were talking to Lank and as he walked toward the kitchen, George directed Lank's attention to something behind him. Lank stopped, looked back, lost his balance and fell. Fortunately the couch broke his fall and he wasn't hurt. Lank admitted this was not the first time he had fallen recently: earlier, while walking toward the kitchen, his telephone rang in the living room. When he stopped and stepped backward to change directions, he fell.

My father often fell in places he was familiar with in and round the home. Falls were due to an assortment of problems: bone spurs, a pinched nerve, poor circulation and the residual effects from his stroke. He really had to concentrate to stand, walk forward and move backwards. When he was walking forward, we learned not to say anything that would cause Lank to look back like "Are you going to take your . . . ?" or "Oh, you forgot . . . . "

To combat Lank's problem with falling, we put in half an hour to forty-five minutes each evening helping him practice: walk forward a few steps, stop and then walk backwards. We went slowly, stressing the importance of not moving quickly when changing directions. We reminded him that people who knew him would know he moved slowly and would wait for him to answer the telephone.

There are two specific surfaces which elderly people find difficult to walk on: grass and thickly padded carpet. When outside, avoid grass or give assistance when grass is inescapable. Where thick carpets are involved, furniture can be strategically placed where someone moving from room to room can rest or balance themselves.

There are a number of concerns with strategic furniture placement: ease of reach, strength and balance of furniture pieces, dangers of falling and so on. These concerns need to be balanced. A therapist once told us she didn't approve of the way our furniture was arranged and stiffly suggested we remove certain pieces she felt were hazardous to Lank. We disagreed. She saw what she had learned in school: furniture clogging pathways. She did not consider our father's need for the independent mobility the chairs and tables provided. What was a hazard to her was a lifeline to him.

It is important to look at the individual situation when arranging furniture and removing obstacles. Removing chairs Lank used to move about the house would be taking away some of his autonomy by limiting his ability to get himself around. No one wants to feel like a prisoner confined to one room in their own home.

Fighting Depression

Depression is a serious problem for the elderly. They are often dealing with compounded losses such as the death of relatives and friends, perhaps also the loss of physical capabilities and limitation of freedom. While listening to and accepting our parents' thoughts on loss helps build and secure a solid trust level, sometimes grief therapy may be necessary to help them with their late year losses.

During Christmas 1993, Lank was experiencing a bad case of "the holiday blues." Remembering past holidays plummeted him into deep depression. Ironically, what precipitated his depression was a visit with my sister Veronica and her son. They spent a week with him between Christmas and New Year's and while their visit thrilled him, their leaving took a big psychological toll. Lank did not want to get out of bed, eat or change clothes.

On the fourth day after my sister's departure, Lank asked me to help him commit suicide. He had been saving sleeping pills because one day he just might want to take the easy way out. Tearfully, we sat together and I validated his feelings by agreeing that killing himself was one option for ending his pain. But I assured him George and I would always be there to care for him. My heart ached for this sad, lonely man as he sobbed uncontrollably. Once he stopped crying, he told me why he wanted to die. Through tears, Lank expressed his desire to see his mother, father, brothers and sister, who were dead. He was tired of living because life was not the same. He said living took too much effort and he was lonely.

I suggested we arrange a trip for him to visit Barbara, my oldest sister, in Alabama. In Alabama he could eat seafood and be warm. He smiled for the first time. We could see if Barbara would drive to Salt Lake City for him since flying was too traumatic. A spark of hope showed in his eyes as we made plans to call Barbara the following day. We talked until the wee hours of the night, when sheer exhaustion caused him to fall asleep. At that immediate time, it didn't matter whether Barbara could make it or not because my motive was to get him to see that other options would make life look less bleak.

The next morning, even though Lank seemed somewhat better, I called a psychologist who specialized in gerontology. She severely reprimanded me for how I dealt with Lank's situation and said I should have institutionalized him. Nevertheless, she suggested I bring Lank to her office where she would evaluate him. I told her Lank would never knowingly go to a doctor for emotional or mental problems and he felt a strong stigma attached to anyone who did. She told me to do whatever it took to get him help, even if it required lying. I refused her help.

For spiritual and emotional support, I contacted Lank's minister and for his depression, medications and physical condition, his doctor. Each offered comfort and suggestions that left Lank with a sense that people cared. Lank's doctor wrote a prescription for two outside walks per day, weather permitting, otherwise an outside ride for fresh air. Because these were written doctor's orders, Lank followed them. Barbara and Veronica were pleased Lank was willing to spend one month with each of them and Lank was looking forward to the trip, giving him reason to do his regular daily routines.

Depression can be handled many ways. Don't be afraid to talk about it. By talking, you may discover a way that is comfortable both to your belief system and your parents' system.

Shopping for Lank's Physician

Just as elderly parents need to trust caregivers, both need to trust their physicians. That means the caregiver has to help "shop around" for the right doctor for their parents' needs. And while most physicians are dedicated, competent and trustworthy professionals, they are people too. Look for that special physician who is compassionate, caring, understanding and appreciative of the parent. Also, you will want a physician who accepts assignment of Medicare patients and is willing to bill secondary insurance companies. Finally, your parent may have prejudices that restrict just who is the right physician.

It's often difficult to find a doctor who accepts new Medicare patients. On top of that, with Lank we also had to contend with his prejudices. That made it very difficult for us to find service providers, whether we were looking for an aide, nurse, therapist or physician. The first time we took Lank to a doctor who was Japanese, Lank immediately told us he wanted another one. What Lank wanted was a white male Anglo-Saxon Protestant. Nobody else would do, at least in the beginning.

We looked to the Physicians' Referral Service where we found another doctor. But we had a communication problem with doctor number two and we stopped using him. We changed doctors for the third time and, while this doctor fit Lank's required pedigree, it was difficult to complete the doctor's visit within three hours because we had to travel in heavy traffic to his office approximately fifteen miles from our home. Although we had already been through a couple of disappointing doctors, we thought surely the percentages would be in our favor now. Doctor number three turned out to be a lemon too. We felt we had entered the Twilight Zone with this third physician.

Lank's first office visit to doctor number three was for a routine check-up. On the second visit, Lank was given a prescription which cost $50 to fill. When we got home, the telephone was ringing. It was doctor number three's receptionist wanting to know what medicine the doctor had prescribed for Lank. When I told her she said the doctor wanted Lank to take something different. I told her we already purchased the expensive medicine. She apologized and suggested we drive back to the doctor's office for free samples to defray the cost. Because we knew Lank's insurance would refund his prescriptions costs at the end of the year, and because I wasn't about to drive that far a second time, I declined her offer. Instead, I asked her to call our pharmacy with the new prescription. A short time later we received a second call, this time from the doctor's nurse. She asked the same questions the receptionist had asked and again we were told not to fill the prescription; she would have the doctor call in another one.

Unbelievable, but that's not all. An entire day passed. Then the doctor called. He wanted to know what prescription his nurse had called in to our pharmacy and I told him. He didn't want Lank to take any medications until he personally called in a prescription. When I hung up the phone, George and I just stared at each other in amazement; it seemed obvious that no one was putting notes in Lank's medical file. Needless to say, we did not have the prescription filled and we never went back to that doctor again. Tough as it was, we went looking for a new physician. Again.

Trust is a key element in any relationship. We kept looking until we found a doctor we and Lank could trust. While physicians one, two and three failed to gain our trust, it is important to note these are isolated cases. Perhaps we've had better luck finding doctors for our other parents because they did not have prejudicial restrictions. As we've previously stated, the vast majority of physicians are dedicated, competent and trustworthy professionals. When you find one, put your trust in that individual until given reason not to. If your parent has prejudices, you probably will have to live with those prejudices. But stay focused and keep looking—the right doctor is out there.

Prejudices can be overcome: Lank's next and final physician was a *woman*. Change is difficult for all of us and especially hard for those who have been set in their ways for as many years as Lank was. Still change became possible for Lank when he realized how hard we were working to provide the kind of doctor he wanted even though our options were few. We showed genuine concern and we talked with Lank about the difficulty of finding a doctor who accepted Medicare.

A major concern for us was finding a doctor whose office was located close enough it wouldn't take a half day to complete a round-trip visit. We had the option of calling Flextrans, a transportation service for the elderly. But while Flextrans might have been an effective way of getting Lank to the doctor, we believed it was an insensitive way to send him. Doctor visits can be frightening, particularly if you can't hear well and are not used to asking questions. Add to those limitations being transported by a stranger in an unfamiliar city and a routine doctor's visit could easily become a traumatic ordeal.

Fortunately for us, the wife of a good friend had recently received her medical degree and was setting up private practice. George called and asked if she accepted assignment of Medicare payments. She did and agreed to take our parents as patients. When we asked Lank, he told us he was concerned about seeing a woman doctor but because he knew what we were going through to find a physician he agreed to give her a try.

Lank's new doctor was beautiful with him and fit our requirements to a tee. Lank's prejudice against having a woman for a doctor went out the window the first time the two of them met. He truly liked her and the embarrassment he thought he would experience with a female physician never became a problem. Once he gave a female doctor a chance, he pleasantly realized women can do more than cook, have children and care for a home. Most obstacles can be overcome given a little time and understanding. Be patient.

Disappointing Professionals

It is important to keep a high profile when any professional, physician, nurse, therapist, aide, hospital or nursing home staff is providing care. A multitude of situations can occur where your presence, your involvement and your willingness to ask questions can help provide a positive outcome. For instance, you may discover a physician has unknowingly written incorrect nursing home admittance orders, or your parents' therapist has a lack of people skills or does not thoroughly understand his or her objectives, or the aide you have brings personal problems to your home, talking always about his or her home life instead of focusing on your parent. By paying attention, staying involved, keeping a high profile, you can spot these or other problems quickly and do something to correct them.

It also is important to know what is going on so your parent's wishes can be protected. This is especially true when they are unable to communicate what they want. At such times, the caregiver must make the decision on behalf of the parent. The responsibility stays with the caregiver; it should never be passed to the doctor. There are legal issues doctors need to address with regard to an individual's right to privacy such as giving medical records and information to someone other than a family member but such issues do not alleviate the frustration that is felt when you see your parent disoriented and you don't know why and can't find out why. Communication with the care team professionals is essential.

Learn as much about each service provider as you can. Watch how they perform their services and ask questions while you watch. Then, if a substitute nurse, aide or therapist is used, see if they do the procedure differently and if they do, ask why. Asking questions and keeping a high profile makes a difference in the quality of care.

One therapist caused a number of problems by overstepping her limits. Once after Lank was discharged from the hospital, a physical therapist was assigned to help him regain his strength. After two visits, without asking George first, the therapist told Lank she wanted George to work with him three times a day with various walking, sitting and standing exercises. Lank believed whatever a medical professional said was gospel, so he took the therapist's suggestion and tried to pin George to times for his daily workouts.

The therapist's approach did not sit well with George. George did not have a problem with helping Lank, but he did have a problem with the therapist committing his time without discussing it with him. He waited until the therapist returned and told her if she wanted him to help Lank, she should discuss it first with him. That way, if he couldn't help, he could make other arrangements without letting Lank down. For her not to give him the option of controlling his own time, he told her, was inconsiderate, inappropriate and unappreciated. Although this was her "first offense," she was the last straw in a long line of disappointing professionals. She apologized and promised that, if in the future, she thought George could be of help, she would come to him before saying anything to Lank.

A short time later the same therapist told us Lank needed a quad cane because it would give him more stability when walking. Rather than have Lank try the cane first, she brought one with her and billed Medicare. Later, a substitute therapist evaluated Lank's physical characteristics and told us a quad cane hindered his mobility and suggested Lank discontinue using it. Lank progressed much faster without the quad cane.

Thus we felt the expenditure for the quad cane was a waste of Medicare funds. Soon after Lank told me the therapist tried to talk him into having bone spurs removed and he was afraid she could force him to do so. We promised Lank that if he didn't want surgery, any surgery, we would support his choice. We had to convince him the therapist could not force surgery on him.

When the therapist told me Lank would not live through the summer I was thrown off guard and deeply concerned when she made her prediction. If she was confident in her forecast, she could be conveying unknowingly to Lank that something was wrong. When I told George what she said, he became livid because we always maintained a positive attitude around Lank and no way was the therapist's prediction positive. We believed the therapist's opinion was outrageous and could negatively affect her care of Lank, that she had overstepped her bounds. George wanted to speak to her in person and when he did, she became argumentative and tried to defend her actions. She was discharged.

Healing Old Wounds and Knowing One's Limitations

I had never confronted my father about the hurt and anger I felt from my childhood. So when he called to ask if he could live with us, I was carrying some heavy baggage I needed to get rid of. I needed to work through those memories and put closure to them forever. It wasn't easy, but over time I learned that by *caring* for him it was possible to *care* for him.

For the first three years Lank lived with us, I mechanically cared for him. While I tended to his needs such as his laundry, shopping and cleaning, it was difficult for me to reach out to him with genuine loving hugs and touches. It was George who filled the void and provided Lank with the hugs and foot rubs. My mechanical care was balanced only by George's sensitivity to both Lank and me. As time passed and our renewed relationship progressed, I began feeling differently about him. I learned to love this man who was my father and I was proud I could express that love by caring for him. Most importantly, Dad felt loved.

My transformation paid off in November 1994 when Dad had been living with us for four years. At this time George's father was also living with us in upstairs quarters. I was working, George was out of town and our cousin Boots was caring for both our fathers when she found my Dad lying on the floor next to his bed. She helped him to his bed and called me. I attempted to call Dad's doctor while Boots called her husband for help at home. Dad's doctor suspected a urinary tract infection and when her suspicion was confirmed, she ordered antibiotics and told us to call her day or night if Dad had further troubles. If necessary she would have him hospitalized.

Dad was incontinent for three days, meaning he could not control bowel or bladder function. While George stayed upstairs with his father, I was downstairs with mine. If either of us needed assistance, we would call the other for help. I turned Dad every two hours to prevent skin break down that could develop into pressure ulcers. Such an injury is usually caused by unrelieved pressure that damages the skin and underlying tissue. Also known as bed sores, pressure ulcers range in severity from mild (minor skin reddening) to severe (deep craters down to muscle and bone). Those bedridden and unable to move may get pressure ulcers in one to two hours. Because the force on the skin is greater when sitting, individuals confined to chairs and unable to move can get pressure sores sooner.

I cleaned Dad and changed the bed every two hours due to his incontinence. I fed Dad and forced him to drink fluids to prevent dehydration. Still, there were no signs of improvement as his physical capabilities kept diminishing. We knew we had to get him on his feet soon because if he stayed in bed much longer, at his age he could lose approximately ten percent of his strength per day. That strength might not ever be regained.

At daybreak on the fourth day, George and I discussed Dad's situation and agreed we could not continue as we were. We had expected Dad's antibiotics to bring improvement within a matter of days. We also believed we were capable of taking care of his incontinence but found "custodial care" required routine checks around-the-clock that could be better handled by multiple caregivers. In other words, we needed a number of family members or a nursing staff and we didn't have either. Dad needed to be in the hospital where he could receive around-the-clock care and intravenous antibiotics which would be more effective. We had done all we could but Dad needed more support so we looked for help. We called his doctor to see what options we had. She advised us to take Dad to the hospital where she would leave orders to have him admitted.

Dad said he understood why I couldn't keep up our current pace any longer and why it was necessary we have him hospitalized. He added: "Will they be as nice to me there as you have been to me?" "Better," I told him. Tearfully, I assured him George and I would make certain they took good care of him. I felt as though my mother was with us that day and I felt she was pleased to see us come so far. Our relationship had truly healed.

Since Dad's condition was uncertain, we called the hospital for transportation. They sent a door-through-door wheel chair van. In non-emergencies, a hospital social worker or discharge planner arranges transportation, generally through a bonded, privately owned member of the National Medical Transportation Association. Door-through-door means the wheelchair bound are transported from the door of their home to the door of the hospital. All states have similar programs and hospitals are aware of what transportation services are available. Cost are approximately $30 plus $1 per mile as opposed to the $600 cost of dispatching an ambulance. This service is a solution for individuals who need more than a bus or taxi but not an ambulance.

Six days after Dad was admitted to the hospital, his doctor suggested having him admitted to a nursing home for rehabilitation. There, a therapist could help him regain his strength while Dad continued to undergo treatment for his infection. Knowing how he felt about being placed in a nursing home, we prepared ourselves to ease any stress Dad was sure to have. We knew we would need to convince him the nursing home was only to be used for his recovery, nothing else. To do that we needed to do our homework.

An Agonizing Path: Nursing Homes and Rehabilitation Support Centers

Nursing home placement of a parent, even for a short period of time, can cause more stress for the adult child than death or divorce. However, choosing a nursing home can be less stressful if you do your homework. Do not chose a facility strictly because it is convenient to your home. Instead, look for a facility that will meet the specific needs of the parent. If the need is for physical rehabilitation, look for a facility that has an in-dwelling physical therapist available at least six days a week. A full-time dietitian should be an intricate part of the facility. Look for staff that are courteous and responsive to patients. Look beyond the facade: many care facilities have been around for years and may look dilapidated but still have all the important services. Above all, involve your parents in the choice of nursing home or care facilities.

You may ask your parent's physician to recommend a facility but be aware there are factors at work that may prevent the doctor from giving the best recommendation. For instance, physicians are more than likely to select a facility where they have privileges and understandably so: it would be impossible for a physician to place patients in all of the homes throughout a city and still maintain a private, family practice.

Also, your physician may not be able to recommend the best facility because he or she has vested interest in that facility. This is more likely to happen in small communities where there are only one or two nursing homes. If a physician has a financial interest in a particular nursing home, Medicare regulations prohibit the doctor from recommending it. However, if your doctor is the staff physician of the nursing home you select, that is a plus but it should not be your number one concern. The general quality of care is more important.

Our experiences have shown that nursing home physicians are very conscientious in working to resolve the problems of the elderly. Meet and question them about their expectations and what goals they have set for your parent, then decide for yourself. Every year a survey of each facility is conducted by the health department; results are available to the public. Any deficiencies against the nursing home will be listed in the report. Ask the nursing home to show you its current report card or contact a state nursing home ombudsman, who is required to have current report cards for all facilities. State ombudsmen should be listed in the state government section of your telephone directory under Aging Services.

Dad's physician recommended three facilities. We weren't comfortable with what we saw after visiting them, so we went looking for another. After visiting a number of institutions, we chose a rehabilitation facility geared to get people back to work, play and life. The therapy program was intense and the atmosphere alive with hope. We told Dad we found a rehabilitation facility where he would work with a therapist to regain lost strength. Once his strength returned, we told him, we would bring him home. Dad was fearful because the facility was far from our home and he thought we would abandon him but he agreed to go after we assured him otherwise. To reassure him and soften his fears, George and I would call one day and visit the next.

In conjunction with the staff, who encouraged family participation, we talked incessantly to Dad about working hard and going home. When the day to discharge him came, his confidence in us as his care managers heightened. As much as he hated therapy, Dad worked hard and we honored our commitment: he was out of the facility in six days and in great spirits. George and I were proud of his efforts toward a speedy recovery as he was of us in getting him back home. Working together as a team made the difference.

Two months later, another emergency prompted another search for a temporary care facility. As Dad recovered, his doctor suggested placing Dad in a rehabilitation facility. George and I thought that was a good idea so we told Dad we were having him moved from the hospital to another facility where he could regain his strength. He readily admitted he was not ready to be released to his apartment.

While Dad was undergoing rehabilitation, we needed to assess whether or not he would still be capable of staying in his downstairs apartment once he completed his therapy. If he were not capable of doing so, we would need to prepare our spare room upstairs and have available whatever assistance would be necessary. We also had a new concern: Dad did not want to go back to the first rehabilitating facility because he felt they had made him work too hard. He wondered if there was somewhere else he could go. We agreed to see what was available. We contacted a nursing home close to our home. I had volunteered there on several occasions. I was very fond of this home and the people who were its administrators. The staff members lived their mission in the care they gave. There were three things we needed to know: Did our doctor have medical privileges at the facility? Was a room available for the next day? Would Dad's stay be covered by Medicare? The answer was yes to all three questions. Furthermore, if Dad was admitted, he would receive one-and-one-half hours of therapy each day, which would seem more reasonable to him than the three hours a day required at the prior facility. There was only one drawback: this was a "nursing home," which had negative connotations to Dad.

That evening, when George and I explained to Dad what type of facility we were considering, his fear about going to a nursing home was evident. We said we would give him all of the information we could concerning the facilities we looked at and he could decide which one he wanted. We told him there was a facility only five blocks from our home and if he chose it, we could visit him every evening and help him with his therapy. George also told Dad he would make sure the therapist at the facility understood our intent to have Dad home as soon as possible. We also reassured him that, as before, if he worked hard he could be released from the facility when he was ready: in three weeks or even three days. It was all up to him. Dad chose the nursing home close to our home.

Dad's transfer to the nursing home had an unexpected effect on me. Despite my regard for this home, when we walked into the building I wondered if I had made a mistake. The halls seemed dark to me and when I saw Dad in the nursing home for the first time, I felt I had betrayed him. I wanted him out of there. I needed to remind myself to stay focused and positive, to remember our goals. George assured me everything was under control and reminded me that since we had already moved Dad to this nursing home we needed to keep a positive outward appearance for him. Also we needed to keep repeating to him how important it was he do the best he could, that he stay focused on his goals. We needed to stress he was not in the same position as the people who lived there. His stay would be only temporary.

Once in the nursing home, it was important for Dad to understand his rights as a patient. For example, at first Dad was not aware he had the right to eat in his room rather than in the dining room. He believed, as do many people his age, that he had to do whatever the nurses told him. We explained what his rights were and that he could stand firm with the staff as to where he wanted to eat. We felt if he stayed in his room, except when he went to therapy, he would stay focused and not get depressed. The nursing staff was very positive and supportive of our goals and they liked visiting with Dad. This made it easier for him to keep focused toward going home.

Dad bounced back in record time, not only physically, but mentally as well. After being in the nursing home for only eight days, he was released. He seemed to be enjoying himself back at home because, once again, he was caring for himself, something he had not been sure he would be able to do.

Major Heart Attack

As mentioned earlier, peculiar behaviors or mannerisms could be warning signs to a major problem. Timing will be important if you are called on to help someone who is experiencing a stroke or heart attack. Prepare now because what you do—or don't do—could mean the difference between life and death. Know beforehand if the person you're caring for wants to live at all cost or wants life and death to take its course. Who will you call if a person is possibly having a heart attack? 911? The physician? A nurse? Fire department? Ambulance service? Family members? Should you try to help by administering CPR or mouth-to-mouth resuscitation? Also know what responsibilities you will have toward your parent, family, friends, work and others. How does your employer's family leave policy work? Will you have sufficient time away from your job to put things in order?

Paying attention helped us help Dad when he again began to show signs of weakness in April 1995. He had fallen on three consecutive days. Although he told us of the falls, he never complained of being injured nor did it appear he had been hurt. Still we started to check on him every two or three hours. On the fourth day, I found Dad lying on his living room floor. He had fallen and was unable to lift himself. He was incontinent and had difficulty completing thoughts. We called his physician and informed her of his condition. She wanted him admitted to the hospital overnight for tests and observation.

Once Dad was settled in his hospital room, George and I went home. Within two hours, we received a call from the charge nurse. Dad was having a massive heart attack. Dad's physician had notified the hospital staff no heroics were to be used. He was only to be kept comfortable and free of pain. George and I spent the next two nights at the hospital and, while there, I contacted my manager at work and was told to concentrate on my father and not worry about my job. He assured me we could work out my schedule later.

The day after Dad's heart attack, reports confirmed only fifteen percent of his heart and kidneys were functioning. He was dying. It was just a matter of time. Because of our timing, Dad was fortunate to be in the hospital before his heart attack happened. If it had happened in his apartment when he was alone, chances are he would have died, slowly and painfully. By paying attention to early warning signs and getting Dad to the hospital early where he was under the watchful eyes of the hospital staff, much of Dad's potential pain and discomfort were eliminated.

The Family Vigil

When an elderly parent is near death, that person's loved ones including his or her caregivers are lucky to have some time to prepare for that death. Preparations can begin as family members congregate at the hospital or the caregiver's home. Family support is invaluable at this time. Primary caregivers should not hesitate asking for help. Caregivers can ask family members to stay with the parent so they can accomplish needed tasks such as preparing the home for the parent's dying process and confirming the family leave policy at work. Family members can alternate time spent at the hospital, staying visible and vocal during this vulnerable time. If the hospital staff does something that makes no sense, ask, "Why are you doing that?" or, "What is the purpose of what you are doing?" or, "How will that benefit my parent?"

Our support system started when I called my sisters to tell them our father had had a heart attack and was not expected to live, it could be hours, days or weeks, but death was imminent. I suggested they take the first available plane to Salt Lake City and asked that they notify relatives of Dad's situation. Meanwhile we had Dad transferred to a private room where our family could gather without interruption. Dad would remain there until the doctors were sure he was stabilized. Then Dad could return home to die just as he had told us he wanted to do.

Since my sisters Veronica and Barbara could stay only one week, I asked them to take turns staying nights with Dad. They could use this time to say their good-byes because both knew they would never again see Dad alive. While I'm not sure they understood my wish that someone stay around the clock with Dad, I was grateful when they agreed to do so. My reasons soon became apparent to them. Just as George and I had defended Dad's well being from aides in the past, my sisters found themselves defending Dad against the physical therapists who wanted to walk him down the hall—right after he had had a devastating heart attack.

The doctor *had* requested a therapist assist Dad with range-of-motion exercises only. Depending on the philosophy of the physician, range of motion for an alert dying person like Dad provides a sense of feeling and touch. Also, the action seems to provide a comfort for the family. If the patient is not alert and not expected to live beyond a week or two, generally no range of motion is recommended. The hospital therapist had misunderstood the doctor's orders and wanted to walk a man who was dying.

During the day our cousins visited with Dad, giving Barbara and Veronica a few hours of relief. Also, Dad's grandchildren called regularly to chat with Pop-Pop, as they called him, and tell their grandfather they loved him. Even though Dad appeared at times to be sleeping or just staring into space, he heard every word we said: Dad answered all the questions we asked him. Since we knew he was listening, we always included him in our conversations.

When Dad's physician was making her rounds, she stopped to introduce herself to our family. While there, without actually saying Dad was going to die, she explained the seriousness of his condition. "People die," she said to Dad, "when the heart and kidneys cease to function. You will be returning home soon, where a nurse will help with your care." Home is where Dad wished to be and by hearing the doctor say this, he knew his wish would come true.

Preparing for Hospice

Hospice is a community nursing service that focuses on dying with dignity. It educates both the caregiver and the dying person about the dying process. Hospice supports families that care for terminally ill people and encourages patients to live the end of their lives in the well known surroundings of their own homes. Hospice offers a wide assortment of services that are covered 100 percent by Medicare. A nurse is available around the clock to assist in pain and comfort control. Once a person is placed on hospice, Medicare pays for all medication; before that point, you pay. Hospice obtains medical supplies, equipment, medicine and assists in every aspect of terminally ill care. It also provides a social worker for the family, after the death, to help them as they grieve.

We made arrangements at the hospital for a hospice nurse to come to our home to assist us with Dad's care once he was settled in. Our failure to get order numbers, the names of persons we spoke to and follow up phone numbers all contributed to a shaky start. Dad was to be released from the hospital by 11 a.m. the following morning. The hospital's transportation van would bring him home where a hospital bed and oxygen supplies were supposed to be waiting for him. The discharge coordinator called at 10:30 a.m. and said the driver was waiting to bring Dad home. I said the driver needed to wait because the bed and oxygen we had ordered had not arrived. When I called the rental company to find out what was going on, they had no record of my order. They promised to check their paperwork and get back to me. Hours passed with no information from the supply company. The discharge coordinator and transportation driver were continually calling, trying to determine when Dad could be released. By late afternoon, someone called and reported our equipment was on the way. When the equipment was finally delivered, we called the hospital and told the transportation driver to bring Dad home. But when the medical equipment driver arrived, he informed us the water container necessary to run the oxygen tank was missing. Dad did not arrive until late afternoon, only minutes after his bed and oxygen were in place.

Within the first hour of his arrival home, though feeling exhausted, Dad was able to eat an ice cream bar, the last thing he was ever to eat. The hospice nurse arrived just moments after he finished and together the four of us discussed comfort and freedom from pain. We could tell when Dad's lungs were filling with fluids because he made a gurgling sound and his breathing became labored. The nurse explained we would be giving Dad Lasix, a water pill which, in essence, would ring him out like a sponge and prevent him from drowning in his own fluids. We were told the time would come when his kidneys 'would stop working: he would go to sleep and die, painlessly, of renal failure.

After the Hospice nurse left, George and I seated ourselves on opposite sides of Dad's bed. George asked Dad if he knew what was happening and Dad said, "The evil spirits are here." Rubbing his hand, I said, "No, God is here. Keep your eyes focused on God." George gently reminded him he was in his own home where he wanted to be when he died. He assured Dad we would not leave him alone and we loved him. George told Dad he had been a good father and provider and assured him he needn't worry about his daughters because they could take care of themselves.

I left a message on Dad's minister's answering machine trying to explain Dad's mental pictures of evil spirits. If Dad had unfinished business, I was hoping his minister would ease his fears. But his minister didn't contact us until it was too late. My priest, however, provided me with certain comforting scripture readings which I hope helped Dad.

Our hospice nurse gave us comfort and the assistance we needed to allow my father to die free of pain and with dignity. Knowing what was happening during the dying process helped us prepare for his inevitable death.

The Way He Died

On Lank's first day home, George and I started an around-the-clock vigil. I read to Dad from the Bible, something he did daily, and together we recited the twenty-third Psalm and said the Lord's Prayer. He didn't actually say the words but moved his lips as I read aloud. George spoke about how glad he was to have known Dad and thanked him for his friendship. He had done a great job bringing up his girls, evident by how they turned out. George read poems and played Dad's favorite cassette tape of old gospel songs by B. J. Thomas.

On the second day, George had to address a very sensitive situation. A cousin was pureeing a large quantity of meat — steak *and* pork chops — for Dad. But Dad was rejecting food and water. For this reason, George delicately explained that the food she was cooking would never be eaten, Dad was dying and we were just making sure he was comfortable and free from pain. By the third day Dad was having difficulty swallowing his medicine and, as the hospice nurse had forewarned us, his body was beginning to twitch excessively. We turned him every two hours to prevent his skin from breaking down into pressure ulcers.

We moistened Dad's mouth and adjusted covers to maintain equal body temperature because while his upper body was perspiring, his legs were cold and he had splotchy red and white skin called mottling, a sign of restricted circulation. His body twitched and his breathing was labored. All the while his lungs gurgled. We contacted the hospice nurse who assessed Dad's condition, then notified the doctor of her findings. We purchased liquid morphine and placed it under Dad's tongue using an eye dropper. When asked to stick out his tongue, he would, letting us know he could still hear us. The morphine immediately reduced the twitching and workload of his heart. Dad hadn't eaten in several days and now he stopped drinking. His output of urine was low and we wondered how long his body could continue without drinking fluids. Nevertheless, since he could hear, we continued to read and talk to him while his favorite music played.

Mid-afternoon of the fourth day I felt his legs and discovered they were cold. While I was trying to restore circulation by rubbing his legs, Sarah, our 16-year-old terrier, suddenly leaped from the floor, to a chair, then onto the bed. She stood starring and sniffing Dad's body, then curled up and laid back against him. Immediately he relaxed.

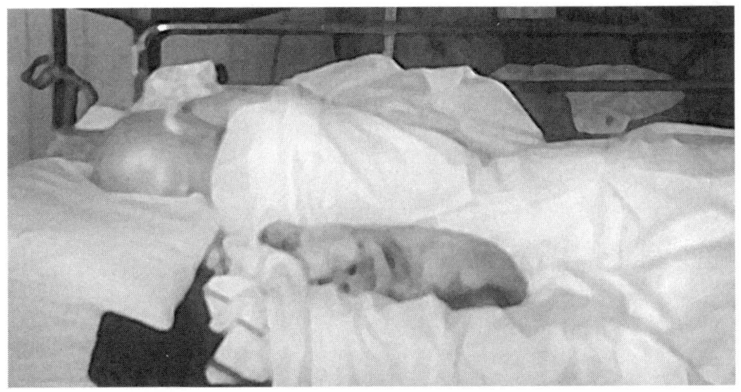

When Dad was healthy, he played with Sarah daily and she never jumped up or sat on his lap. Nevertheless she seemed to have a sixth sense of what was happening and her presence had a soothing affect. As Sarah lay there, Dad's breathing was getting shallow and periodically we needed to check to see if it had stopped. Because repositioning at this time caused him discomfort, we waited until morning before we turned him.

On the fifth day the hospice nurse came to our home to check on Dad. While standing at the bed discussing his condition, George said, "I think this is it." Dad's breathing was extremely shallow, decreasing in strength and length. George took one of Dad's hands and I took the other. As Dad took his last breath, we said, "Good-bye." As George and I held each other tearfully, the nurse turned off Dad's oxygen. The room went completely quiet. It was then I felt the impact of my father's death.

The easiness with which Dad died made it easier for us to accept. Knowing that we gave him the best care we could during the most vulnerable time of his life gave us great satisfaction. Having the knowledge and professional assistance we had made this experience comfortable and rewarding. It was rewarding because we had been able to do for this once-domineering, controlling individual what he could not do for himself. It was comfortable because we knew what we had done for this now kind and elderly gentleman was done with love and understanding. Dad died May 15, 1995.

Watching someone die is not easy. If you care for an elderly person, knowing what, when and how to give care will help ensure your parent dies in comfort, free of pain and with dignity. Imagine what the body and mind experience as the final stages of life pass. Being there before a death and watching someone die, you are witnessing a transformation everyone will make. You are confronted with your own mortality.

The Final Steps

Shortly before the morticians arrived, as a final chance to care for Dad, we washed and creamed his body, dressed him in his pajamas, placed his teeth in his mouth and put his glasses on his face—he was ready to go.

Because of how mobile our society is today, it is rare to find extended family members living in the same geographical area. Thus many elderly parents who move into children's homes come from a different state. They worry about getting back when they die. A funeral agreement may ease some of this fear.

An out-of-state, pre-paid funeral agreement can work smoothly. Dad had a pre-paid funeral agreement in Pennsylvania. George called the Harrisburg funeral home. All he had to do was provide the name of a mortuary in Salt Lake and they would do everything else. The funeral home made arrangements to have Dad's body flown to Harrisburg, Pennsylvania, and once there, they would proceed with the burial agreement. Since Dad had already paid for everything but his flight back to Harrisburg, the only expense we incurred was a $400 airline ticket. The funeral home billed us for this charge only after fulfilling their part of the burial agreement.

When someone dies at home, do not call 911. Instead contact the doctor, hospice nurse, community home care agency, mortuary or police: all are authorized to pronounce a person dead. The mortuary will submit the death certificate to the family physician. The doctor will certify cause of death, sign and submit the certificate to the Office of Vital Statistics where you obtain certified death certificates of the deceased. The cost is minimal. Because various businesses such as airlines, funeral homes, insurance companies and creditors require proof of death, obtain at least five certified certificates.

When Dad died, I contacted my sisters and we collectively made arrangements for his funeral. Veronica organized the funeral service and placed an obituary in the Harrisburg newspaper. She notified everyone of the date and time of the funeral. George asked the airlines for a bereavement fare for those who needed to travel on short notice to attend a family member's funeral. One of the certified death certificate was required to get this fare. George coordinated Barbara's travel time with ours. All she had to do was call and make reservations compatible with ours. The distance from the airport to Harrisburg was significant so whoever drove could pick all of us up at once and avoid two trips. The services were held and, at his request, Dad was dressed in a blue pin-stripped suit. His good friend and favorite minister delivered his eulogy. If it was possible for Dad to have been watching his funeral from above, there is no question he would have been both shocked and elated because that gathering would have surpassed his every expectation.

The Aftermath

We realized once Dad was dead and buried that we had to contend with both our grieving *and* with the aftermath of his death. For example, we had to notify Social Security of his death. We had to sort through statements from healthcare providers, forms from insurance's companies and Medicare EOMB notices. After all insurance claims were paid, if a small balance was left, we reported Dad's death to the providers and notified them that he left no estate. The providers would then write off the remaining balance.

During the latter part of August we received an EOMB notice addressed to the "Estate of M F Albert." This document is reproduced on the following page. When we looked at the first page in a box located in the upper right side titled "the summary of this notice," we discovered for five days rental of medical equipment, the total amount of the original bill was $832.40. This figure seemed pretty high so we began to dig through the notice. Under Services and Services Codes, we discovered that one oxygen concentrator and one portable gaseous O_2 canister had been double billed (see arrows on document). It appeared Dad's estate was responsible for the extra $418.34.

The bill itemized charges for various rental equipment. Lettered notes on the right side of the itemization section correspond to billing explanations located on page 2 of the notice. *Code f* indicated the estate was not responsible for this charge, conflicting with the earlier information. We contacted the rental company and had them correct the problem.

We are disturbed by how Medicare's payment schedule worked, especially in Lank' case. On May 10, 1995, the medical supply company delivered one hospital bed, one commode chair detached, one commode chair fixed, one oxygen concentrator and one portable gaseous O_2 canister. At the time we ordered these supplies, we had no idea what was needed or for how long we would use the items — six months, six weeks, or six days.

The Medicare bill, under "more details about this notice," indicated the approved amount included payment for all covered stationary oxygen equipment, contents and accessory items for an entire rental month. In simple language, Medicare does not prorate or just pay for the days the supplies are used. Even though the equipment and supplies were used for only

THIS IS NOT A BILL
Explanation of Your Medicare **Part B** Benefits

ESTATE OF
M F ALBERT
1234 ANY STREET
SALT LAKE CITY, UT 84000-0000

Summary of this notice dated August 16, 1995		
Total charges:	$	832.40
Total Medicare approved:	$	483.06
We paid your provider:	$	386.45
Your total responsibility:	$	418.34

Your Medicare Number is: 111-11-1111A

Your provider accepted assignment

Details about this notice (See the back for more information.)

BILL SUBMITTED BY: ABC MEDICAL EQUIPMENT
Mailing address: 0000 Main Street, SLC, UT 84000

Dates	Services and Service Codes	Charge	Medicare Approved	See Notes Below
	Control number: 00000-0000-00-000			
May 10, 1995	1 Hosp bed semi-electr w/ matt Rental (E0000-AAAA)	$ 147.20	$ 147.20	a,b
May 10, 1995	1 Commode chair stationary det Rental (E0000-AAAA)	16.74	16.74	a,b
May 10, 1995	1 Oxygen concentrator 2-3 lite Rental (E0000-AAAA)	273.22	273.22	c,b
May 10, 1995	1 Portable gaseous O2 Rental (E0000-AAAA)	48.51	45.90	d
May 10, 1995	1 Commode chair stationary fxd (E0000-AA)	25.00	0.00	e,f
	Control number: 00000-0000-00-000			
May 10, 1995	1 Oxygen concentrator 2-3 lite Rental (E0000-AAAA)	273.22	0.00	g
May 10, 1995	1 Portable gaseous O2 Rental (E0000-AAAA)	48.51	0.00	g
	Total	$ 832.40	$ 483.06	

Notes:

a Monthly rental payments for this item can continue for up to 15 months from the first rental month or until the equipment is no longer needed, whichever comes first.

(continued on next page)

IMPORTANT: If you have questions about this notice, call CGLIC toll free at 1-800-899-7095 or see us at 2 Vantage Way, Nashville, Tenn. You will need this notice if you contact us.

To appeal our decision, you must WRITE to us before FEB 16, 1996LIC P. O. Box 690, Nashville, TN 37202.

See #2 on the back. (000-0005439)

M F ALBERT Page 2

Your Medicare Number is: 111-11-1111A

More details about this notice

b The approved amount is the provider's actual charge for this service.

c The approved amount includes payment for all covered stationary oxygen equipment, contents and accessory items for an entire rental 37 37month.

d The approved amount is based on the fee schedule.

e Medicare cannot pay for this because your provider used an invalid or incorrect procedure code and/or modifier for the service you received. Please ask your provider to resubmit the claim with the valid procedure code and/or modifier.

f You are not responsible for this charge.

g No certification of medical necessity was received for this equipment.

Here's an explanation of this notice:

Of the total charges, Medicare approved	$ 483.06	The provider agreed to accept this amount. See #4 on the back.
Your 20%	- 96.61	We pay 80% of the approved amount; you pay 20%.
The 80% Medicare pays	$ 386.45	**You have already met the deductible for 1995.**
Medicare owes	$ 386.45	
We are paying the provider	$ 386.45	
Of the approved amount	$ 483.06	
Less what Medicare owes	- 386.45	
Net responsibility	$ 96.61	
Plus charges Medicare does not cover	+ 321.73	You are responsible for these denied charges.
Your total responsibility	$ 418.34	The provider may bill you for this amount. If you have other insurance, the other insurance may pay this amount.

IMPORTANT: If you have questions about this notice, call CGLIC toll free at 1-800-899-7095 or see us at 2 Vantage Way, Nashville, Tenn. You will need this notice if you contact us.

To appeal our decision, you must WRITE to us before FEB 16, 1996 LIC P. O. Box 690, Nashville, TN 37202.

See #2 on the back. (000-0005439)

five days, Medicare paid their portion for the entire thirty day contract, less the twenty percent deductible for which Dad's estate was responsible. Perhaps this is another reason why Medicare has financial problems.

Read and understand the *Explanation of Medicare Part B Benefits* notice. Contact the service providers and have them explain what you don't understand. When in doubt, ask questions. Monitor the billing system even after someone dies.

Peaceful Endings

By spending the last years of his life with us, the door was opened for a new friendship between George and Lank. Dad enjoyed a home complete with family. He was not alone and he felt loved. He reflected on both the bad and the good times of his life, sharing with us his joys and giving us a number of lessons.

As I recall my father's last five days of living, I find the opportunity he gave us was highly rewarding because he not only allowed us to witness the most private part of his life, but he let us participate in it as well. That participation was enhanced because we knew we could keep him comfortable and help him live his remaining time in dignity and free of pain.

My father and I first came to terms with each other, then developed the father-daughter relationship that had eluded us earlier in our lives. I received the inner peace that comes from investing time and energy toward the belief that something positive could come from so many hurt-filled years. The love George and I share grew deeper as we worked through the daily challenges of eldercare and building a new relationship with Dad. George and I move forward with more knowledge of aging and with respect for life and for death as well. This experience would serve us as we continued the eldercare journey with George's parents.

George's Father

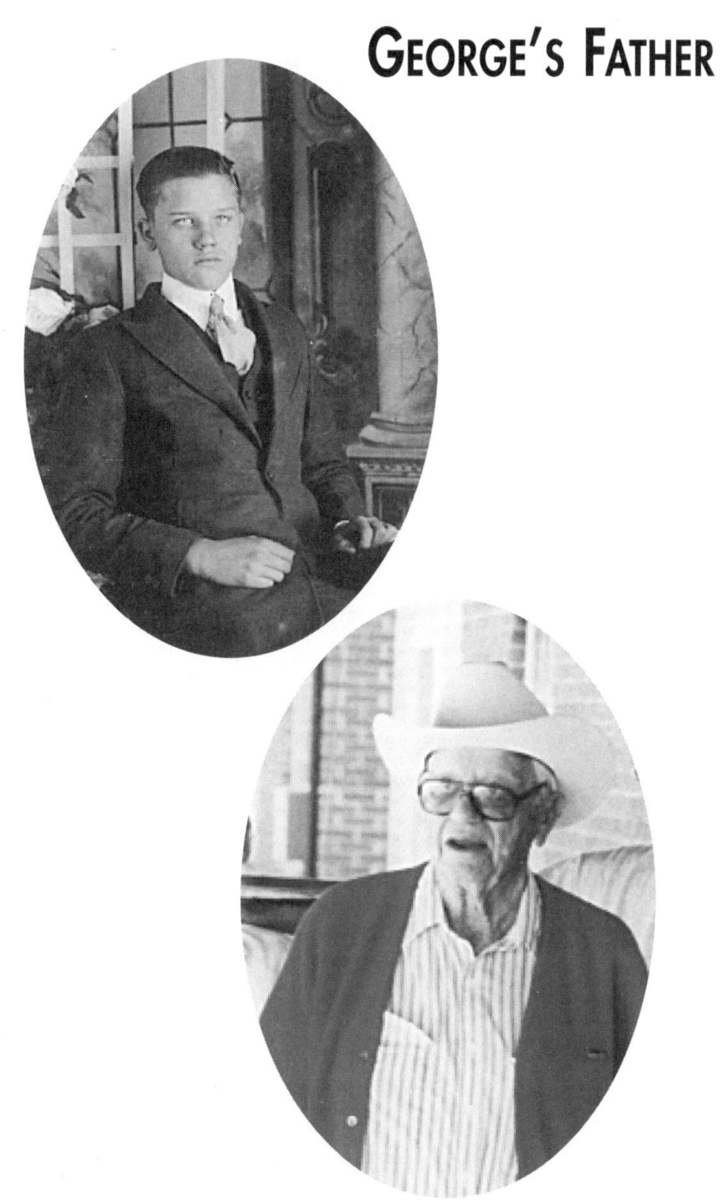

Hardyn Gwen Watson

July 9, 1904 — December 21, 1996

My parents, Hazel and Hardyn Watson, were married July 18, 1931. During the second year of their marriage, my brother Byron was born and eleven months later, I came along. Hardyn worked as a brakeman and as a switchman for Kennecott Copper Corporation's railroad. He worked during the Great Depression and after thirty-seven years of service, he retired at age sixty-five. A few years after his retirement, after forty-three years of marriage, Hardyn and Hazel divorced and went their separate ways. Hazel stayed in the Salt Lake City home where we grew up while Hardyn moved from Salt Lake back East where he had grown up: he moved into an eleven story senior citizens' apartment complex located on the banks of the Ohio river, only an hour from Eby, Kentucky where his sister still resided in the home where he was born.

When Hardyn first started his family, he thought of himself as being "tough" and was determined to make his sons "tough" also. As Byron and I grew, Dad became a stern disciplinarian, sometimes predictable, sometimes not. Like many of the men he worked with, Hardyn had little formal education. Characteristic of the times—The Great Depression—men did whatever was necessary to put food on the table and shelter over their family's heads even if this meant they had to steal to survive. Hardyn and his friends thought of themselves as strong, "macho" men. Their philosophy on rearing children was that if children are good, never acknowledge it but if children are bad, punish them.

During our adolescent years Dad ruled our home with an iron fist and everyone was afraid of him. Years later, through reading and studying social behaviors, I realized Dad carried on the way he did because the pressures to put food on the table were great and he had never been taught how to cope with pressure. Dad would react to pressure with violence. Since he was never taught a different response, he never learned that his type of anger was inappropriate, that he was misdirecting his anger towards his sons instead of recognizing we had no control over the economic conditions of the times. He would go into a rage over a minor infraction—not mowing the lawn, forgetting to take the garbage out. His anger was vented on his son's backs with a razor strap. He never vented anger by going for a walk or talking things out with his wife. He was completely reactive.

As he aged, however, Dad mellowed and violent behavior was no longer part of who he was. Dad changed from a tough disciplinarian to a kind old man. He exhibited a genuine interest in my family and Byron's family and demonstrated his care for us and his grandchildren in action and deed. Even though he lived in Ohio, some 1,500 miles away, our relationships grew.

As Dad moved into his late seventies, he had many friends and family in Ohio and Kentucky who loved him dearly. But unfortunately when he started to need continual assistance, the people he wanted to be with could not care for him, could not because most were elderly and dealing with medical problems themselves.

We saw this transformation in our father. Hopefully, if you witness a similar transformation in your parents, you will have empathy for what that person has lived through. Then perhaps you can give comfort to and have compassion for your parent's plight. You can give them the opportunity to live the rest of their lives with dignity.

Having a Long-Distance Emergency Support System

A support system is particularly important for older parents who live by themselves out of state. Support can be given by a friend, relative, neighbor or church member who can regularly check on a loved one in case a medical emergency suddenly develops.

On October 20, 1992, Nellie, a family friend who lived in Dad's senior complex telephoned to say she had found Dad in his apartment, semiconscious, incoherent and unable to stand. Nellie called 911 for my 88-year-old father and notified Dad's physician that Dad was on his way to the hospital. I telephoned Dad's doctor in Wheelersburg, Ohio. The doctor explained Dad had been admitted to the hospital where he was being given antibiotics for a urinary track infection. Everything would be fine, he said, and there was no cause for worry. Furthermore, since Dad's situation was not life-threatening, he saw no reason for me to come to Ohio.

I telephoned Dad every day he was in the hospital and then I would call my brother, Byron, who lives in Tampa, Florida, to discuss Dad's condition and situation. Byron was also calling every day to let Dad know we both supported him.

On the seventh day, a Saturday, I called the hospital and asked the operator to ring Dad's room. An aide handed Dad the phone and for the first time since his admission he was incoherent and unable to stay focused on our conversation. I was not certain but I had a feeling he didn't know who I was. Worried, I terminated our call and immediately telephoned my brother and explained to him what had happened. Byron told me he would call to see if Dad sounded the same to him and would get back to me as soon as he discovered anything. When Byron called back, he agreed there definitely appeared to be a problem. I told him I would call Dad's doctor to find out what had happened and what was being done to correct the problem. When I called, I was told the doctor was on call for the weekend so I asked his answering service to have him return my call. He never did.

I called Dad again the first thing the following morning. Once again, Dad babbled incoherently. The nurse in charge told me she had checked with the weekend nurse, aides and therapist and no one seemed to know why his behavior was so strange. I expressed my concern and told the nurse that it sounded to me as though he might have had a stroke. She said she couldn't say one way or the other but she would have the doctor get in touch with me when he made his rounds. I wasn't about to wait that long. I called the doctor's office for a second time. He still had not checked in so once again I asked the lady with the answering service to have the doctor call me.

Talk about frustration. The doctor finally returned my call Monday at noon, forty-eight hours after I first called him. He said he had left orders for the hospital staff to walk Dad every morning. I was completely surprised by the doctor's candor when he told me he believed Dad's problem was caused by the fact that no one had followed his orders and for the entire weekend Dad had just lain there in bed. The doctor informed me that the staff was hesitant to walk Dad because he was such a large man—Dad weighed approximately 225 pounds. Remember that ten percent of one's body strength is lost for twenty-four hours of lying in bed. I told the doctor if the hospital staff could not find someone to walk Dad then I would personally fly out to Ohio and see his orders were followed. If I had to be the one helping Dad walk, then so be it. I also believed once I saw Dad I would be better able to evaluate his condition. After numerous long distance calls from Salt Lake to Ohio, I still didn't know what the doctors and nurses were talking about. Byron and I needed to see with our own eyes if Dad could or could not stand and walk without assistance, to determine whether there were specific needs we could address to improve his present condition.

I called my brother and we arranged to travel to Ohio immediately. When we walked into his room, Dad seemed to know who we were but we couldn't understand a thing he was saying because he was speaking in a broken, jabbering, babbling way. Despite what the hospital staff had said, I still felt he had had a stroke. (We later found out he had had approximately five mini-strokes while in the hospital.)

Dad was doing a tremendous amount of hallucinating and neither Byron nor I had any idea why. He would lift his head from the hospital bed and just stare straight at the wall. Then suddenly his eyes would begin to jump, first up and down, then from side to side. It was as if he were watching something happening in his room that we were unable to see. At times when I was standing in front of him he would stare at the zipper on my coat and then very slowly reach out with his forefinger and rub the zipper ever so lightly. That strange stare never left him.

Byron and I were concerned and we needed answers. We met with Dad's physician to discuss what course of treatment the doctor planned to pursue and what he thought was wrong with Dad. He told us he couldn't be sure of the cause but he had seen other patients with similar conditions; sometimes they snapped out of it and sometimes they didn't. He said there was no way to tell what would happen. The only thing we could do was wait and see but for the moment he believed it would be best if we considered placing Dad in a nursing home.

Because Dad's friend and neighbor informed us of his medical problem, we were able to follow up immediately. Nellie supported both Dad and his children by keeping us informed. Byron and I supported each other by telephoning Dad at different times of the day, then sharing our impressions with each other. We were Dad's daily support by phone. We also stayed in contact with the medical staff on his behalf. With Dad and

Nellie in Ohio, Byron in Florida and me in Utah, the phone became our lifeline for Dad.

LOOKING FOR A NURSING HOME IN UNFAMILIAR TERRITORY

Placing a parent in a convalescent home near you, even temporarily, can be distressing for that parent who may feel abandoned. But consider the distress a parent must feel when being placed in a nursing home in another state; after a short time you return to your home, leaving the parent to wonder if you will ever be able to return. Even though your parent is institutionalized in another state, there are things you can do to reduce his or her distress. Call daily. Arrange for friends to visit. Check with medical staff often.

It is extremely important—for your parent's welfare and your peace of mind—that you find the best nursing home available for your parent's special needs. Do your homework.

Our doctor believed it would be best if we considered placing Dad in a nursing home where he would have around-the-clock care and skilled therapists to work with him. He suggested we consider a convalescent center in Dad's hometown, not because it was close to where Dad lived, but because he believed it to be the best one available. The doctor also suggested we visit other facilities to be able to make comparisons.

At the time, my brother and I did not know about the report cards issued by the Health Department. We relied on the doctor's advice to visit other facilities in and around Wheelersburg, then check out the one he recommended. After what turned out to be a disappointing search we finally called the convalescent center our doctor suggested and made an appointment to meet with its administrators.

We spoke with staff, aides and a few patients and found the nursing home to be first class. Each shift had one licensed practical nurse and two to three aides for every three to four patients. There were two registered nurses available at all times. The center was exceptionally clean and fresh smelling and everyone appeared happy and enthusiastic about working there. Because of the skillful and individual attention we observed between the staff and patients, we knew Dad would be in the care of professionals who had the expertise to rehabilitate him. We also felt the staff would see to Dad's personal needs such as assistance to the bathroom, fresh water, someone to talk to and people who would walk him.

It was important to move quickly in getting our father the best possible care. He had been in bed too long and his condition would only get worse without intense physical therapy. Dad's physician said he would sign his release papers for the next day and we should return to the hospital and gather up his personal belongings so he would be ready for discharge the following morning. Also, he said we should contact the hospital's social worker who was responsible to help us get Dad admitted to the convalescent center.

If you are located in the state where your parent is institutionalized, staying visible and vocal is easy. When you live out of state, visibility becomes more difficult; however, you can still make your ongoing interest known with phone calls and the help of friends in the distant location. You need to set up a support system of family, friends, neighbors and church members. We cannot stress enough the importance of this community involvement. When you call your parent, show your support with encouragement. Let him or her know when you will return, then keep your commitment. Last, not least, express your love to your parent.

Phone the charge nurse at the facility and contact the family physician directly to secure current information on how your parent is progressing. Ask for suggestions of what you can do to help.

Keep in touch with your support team. Remember to thank them for their gift of time and caring.

The Miracle

When Byron and I returned to the hospital, we met with the social worker. She said the hospital could start preparing for Dad's release and his transportation to the center. Shortly after leaving her office, both Byron and I were in Dad's hospital room making small talk when Byron decided to go outside and have a cigarette. While Byron was gone I walked over to Dad's bed and sat down next to his side. I placed my face up close to his and looked straight into his blank, empty eyes and said, "Dad, we're taking you out of this hospital. You're going to a home to convalesce." As I said the word "home," I detected a movement in his eyes I hadn't seen before.

I repeated what I had just said and I received the same response to the word "home," but this time the eye movement was more pronounced. Again I repeated the words and once again I received a stronger response on the word "home." His eyes would roll and I could tell he knew what "home" meant. It appeared he was trying to snap out of his trance-like state so he could understand all of what I was saying. I felt like ET in the movie *Extra Terrestrial,* pointing toward the heavens and repeating, "Home . . . Home . . . Home." The little boy just stares in awe as he suddenly understands what ET is saying.

Suddenly, after not speaking coherently for almost a week, Dad asked, "When?" "Tomorrow morning," I responded. His eyes were jumping all over the room as he fought to clear his head and focus on what I was saying. He repeated, "Tomorrow morning?" "Yes!" I shouted. I started telling him what our plans were and since he had just come out of some kind of trance and was talking to me as if we had been involved in some kind of discussion, I went along with him and conversed in the same nonchalant manner. Calmly, I spoke to him as though we had been talking ever since I had arrived in Ohio.

By the time my brother returned, Dad and I were talking about leaving the hospital and going home. When my brother walked into the room and saw us talking, his jaw fell about a foot and he asked, "What the hell has happened?" I simply replied, "Dad and I have been talking about his leaving the hospital and going to a convalescent HOME." Byron was in shock because he had been mentally preparing himself for Dad's death; he was by no means preparing for the possibility of long-term care.

Byron and I stayed most of that evening with Dad, then finally had to tell him we would see him in the morning. The next day was going to be busy. Dad wanted to know exactly when we would be back and we assured him it would be early. We had no idea what the next day would bring. Would Dad be happy that he was out of the hospital or mad because he was in a *nursing home?*

My brother and I questioned each other when we decided without his input to have Dad admitted to a nursing home. Were we doing what was best for Dad? Or what was best for ourselves? We also wondered what he would say or think when we told him of our plans after the fact. How would he respond to our actions? How would he feel if we didn't tell him of our intentions and simply delivered him to the nursing home by ambulance? We believe we made the decision we did because we both wanted to provide Dad with the best possible opportunity to recover from his stroke. We knew if he was going to be rehabilitated, this convalescent center was the place for him to do it.

When you take on the responsibility to make decisions for parents, know that to fulfill their wishes you may be confronted with deciding how and where they will live, be it with you or in a nursing home. You may find yourself questioning your motives. Are they selfish or self-less? Such self-evaluation should be used to help the decision-making process. Making such decisions are not easy. But when you make a decision, stand behind it and don't walk away.

THE ROAD TO RECOVERY: TRIALS AND TRIBULATION

Sure enough, the next morning when we entered Dad's room, he said angrily, "I thought you said I was going home." I responded, "We said you were going to a *nursing* home to convalesce and that's what you need to do. But it's up to you. You're weak now and unable to walk. As soon as you can get on your feet and do the things you were able to do before your stroke, you will go home." He responded, "I can too walk," to which I replied, "Then show us." He tried with all his might to stand, but once he realized what we said was true, he never gave us a hard time about being at the nursing home.

With Dad now settled in and hopefully on the road to recovery, Byron and I returned to our homes. We told Dad we had to leave Wheelersburg and promised him we would call everyday. I told him I would be back in a few weeks. If he wanted to be released from the nursing home when I returned, he would have to work hard with the therapists to regain his strength. Giving him a reassuring hug, seeing tears well up in his eyes, I told him when I returned I wanted him to be in tip-top shape.

When I returned to Salt Lake City, I told Emily that my brother and I intended to wait until after Thanksgiving before we went back to Ohio. But after being home for only two days, I told her I felt guilty about leaving Dad by himself for two weeks, maybe three. Emily agreed I shouldn't wait to go back. She insisted on going with me. We didn't want to take any chances that he might feel abandoned and slip back to where he had been before, hallucinating and incoherent.

Getting time off from work might have been an obstacle in returning to Ohio so soon. But we were lucky. I could arrange affairs in my business to leave for a short time. Emily contacted her boss, explained what had happened and asked if she could have time off to help me with my father. Emily's boss, was great. He told her not to worry and to do whatever she felt was necessary to get Dad back on his feet, and to keep him posted on how well Dad was doing. Everyone at Emily's office, from top management down to her immediate boss, were very supportive.

When we arrived at the nursing home, Dad was ecstatic to see us. We found him walking the halls with his physical therapist who said he was progressing quite well. He also informed us that everyone liked working with Dad and mentioned the nurses had nick-named him "Old Blue-Eyes." I asked about Dad's hallucinations and was told he continued to have some but they had decreased since he'd first arrived at the center.

That evening Emily and I took Dad to the dining room. While we were sitting at the table, I noticed Dad's attention had suddenly focused to something that was apparently on the wall. His eyes were fixed and he had that same blank stare as before. Then suddenly he pointed at whatever it was he saw on the wall and said, "Look! Did you see that? A red fox! It ran right across that open field. God, I haven't seen one of them in years." I merely agreed with him that it was unusual to see a red fox in this geographical area and never mentioned it again. Somehow it made me feel better, however, to think that when Dad had been staring blankly at the walls and ceiling he was actually seeing something he appeared to enjoy. The idea that Dad was seeing something was more appealing to me than the thought that he was in a void, a nonthinking, nonfeeling state. Later on, when I asked Dad about this period of time, he told me he could not remember any of it.

Dad had been in the center for only ten days and his improvement was very encouraging: we hoped to have him back in his own home soon. We asked the nurse in charge if we could take Dad out for a few hours and she said yes, for as long as we wanted. We told her there was a possibility we would go to his sister's home for Thanksgiving and if he did well, we would probably stay overnight.

So on Thanksgiving we took Dad to his sister Ruby's house and since he was moving like his old self, we ended up taking him back to his apartment rather than to the nursing home. Because officially Dad had not been released from the nursing home, Emily and I stayed with him at his apartment for one week. That week gave us ample time to evaluate how he would get along once we left. We made sure he did everything for himself that he would have to do once we were gone. As soon as we were confidant he would be able to maintain his Activities of Daily Living (ADLs)—bathing, dressing, and undressing himself, preparing his own meals, taking the right medicine at the right time and so on—it would be OK for us to return to Salt Lake City.

The road to recovery requires an investment of time and energy for both parent and caregiver. It also requires a belief in family and in family members working together.

Putting Together a More Extensive Support System

The senior citizens' apartment complex where Dad lived was a perfect place for him to return to after a stroke because his apartment offered safe surroundings with little, if any, chance of injury. Once he was home, we started organizing Dad's support system. We found he was not eligible for home-delivered meals because he could walk to the microwave and heat a dinner. So to help with meal times we had one of his neighbors take him to a senior center for lunch. This type of active involvement also provided him with social contact that kept his spirits high.

We also investigated the senior companion program. This program is funded by a number of federal and state agencies who then pay lower-income, able-bodied elderly people to serve as companions to disabled older people. Senior companions work four hours a day, five days a week and the hourly stipend they receive for their service is not subject to taxation. We asked for a senior companion for Dad but knew there could be a waiting list of two years or more. We felt that since Dad had so many friends, relatives and neighbors willing to check on him and provide transportation, we would have no trouble setting in motion a dependable support system for him without having to call on Senior Companion Services.

To help establish Dad's support system and to prevent overlapping or redundant care, we asked specific people to do specific tasks. Each person was happy to oblige. Dad's physician added to the support system by writing orders for a Medicare-covered physical therapist to visit Dad regularly three times a week and for a home health aide to standby-assist to watch to ensure he was safe from falling while showering and dressing.

Once Dad's support system was in place we had him officially released from the nursing home and we returned to Salt Lake City while he remained in Ohio where he was able, with some assistance, to take care of himself. Our decision to have Dad released proved to be correct and he was pleased. He left the convalescent center, never to return, after only ten days.

Dad had no memory of his time in the hospital and the first few days at the nursing home. He never felt comfortable talking about this time lapse. Because in the end he was able to go back to taking care of himself in his own apartment, the experience gave him a reservoir of confidence in our decision-making on his behalf.

Questions for the Long-Distance Caregiver

Many things need to be done when a parent has been stricken with a life-threatening illness and the outcome is uncertain. The situation is further complicated when the parent is living hundreds, even thousands of miles away. We asked ourselves many questions during Dad's illness, questions that are important for anyone in a similar situation to consider. Some of the questions will also apply to the close-by caregiver.

Will we understand the doctor's medical treatment plan well enough to make appropriate medical and therapeutic decisions on behalf of our parent, or will we make mistakes out of confusion, ignorance and distress?

The physician is the key player in this question. We asked numerous questions about our father's treatment plan and when we didn't understand what the doctor was saying, we asked him to continue to explain until we did. We asked questions such as, "Is the treatment more life-threatening than the current condition?" "What is the worse case scenario if he does not have it done?" "What are the advantages of having it done?" "What could his quality of life be if he has it done?" "What could his quality of life be if he does not have it done?" "Are there options in medications?" "What about side effects?" "If he were your father, what would you do?" These types of questions helped us select a course of treatment for our father.

Have we notified everyone we should of our parent's illness?

Rather than trying to call all our relatives and friends by ourselves, we contacted those family members who had been most concerned and requested they contact additional family and friends. Asking for help in this situation allowed us to concentrate on Dad's needs and our preparation for being with him.

What options are available when the emergency purchase of an airline ticket is necessary?

If the distance is so great that it is necessary to fly, the cost of the airline ticket will add greatly to the total expenses. We knew we would have to purchase the ticket regardless of cost. If time had allowed us, we might have purchased a super-saver ticket for which payment would have had to be made fourteen days in advance. We did not have the flexibility to do this, but we still took the time to call each airline to see what was available. As it turned out we had no options because when we purchased our tickets we were leaving for Ohio the next day so we had to pay regular fare.

If we leave now will we need to return soon and stay longer, at increased expense?

The main reason our timing in going to Ohio was so good was because of our communication with Dad's physician and nurses. We were well-informed about his condition because we made daily phone calls to the doctor's office and the nurses' station on his floor at the hospital.

If we wait longer, will we have waited too long?

Again, keeping in close touch with the medical staff is key. If the physician had said, "Come now," then obviously we would have left instantly. Since he suggested that things were under control, we waited. This kept costs down and reduced our time away from work. We understood the physician was only human and we had to rely on our own best judgment to make the final decision.

What will happen with our jobs if we take time off to care for an elderly parent?

I am self-employed and, within reason, I do pretty much as I wish. I'm not able to take off for long periods of time and let my company run itself but I do have flexibility. Emily works for a major corporation and her situation is entirely different. She had to discuss the situation with her boss, find out what the family leave policy was and what company boundaries she would need to work within. American

Express in general, and Emily's manager in particular, were very supportive in working with her when she needed time off to commute from Salt Lake to Ohio.

Fortunately it looks like the flexibility Emily's employer gave us in terms of time off for eldercare may be the wave of the future. An Associated Press article in a September 1995 issue of our local paper reported that twenty-one of the nation's largest companies had announced an unprecedented $100 million, six-year effort to improve child- and elder-care for their employees in communities across the country. The size of this commitment reflects the growing role of women in the labor force and the absence of government aid for working people with children or elderly relatives.

Today, when we look back, we wouldn't change the way we handled our responsibility as long-distance caregivers for my father. There were tough times when we were uncertain when to go and there were scary times when we were uncertain of what was truly happening but because we went with the attitude, "What is best for Dad is what we will do," the experience was rewarding for all of us.

Bringing Long-Distance Caregiving Closer to Home

When my brother and I initially identified Dad's needs and discovered we would have to go back and forth to Ohio to help him, we didn't realize how much more expensive, time-consuming, frustrating and painful it would be to do long-distance caregiving than caring for someone who lives in the same town. For example, we found over the years that if Dad needed to have any kind of operation it was easier for us to have him fly to Salt Lake City and have it here. If he stayed in Ohio to have his operation, we would have to take more time off from work to fly to Ohio to be with him. Also, depending on where the hospital was located in relation to his home, our living quarters for the duration of his hospital stay sometimes wound up being a motel. Also, sometimes we had to buy more than one airline ticket because we might have to leave Ohio before Dad's medical condition was resolved and come back at a later date. Having to deal with the expense and time made the situation more frustrating.

In our case, my brother and I were reimbursed for our expenses because Dad had money in savings. Because of the way our families relate to one another, we would have been able to give Dad the same care because Byron and I would have absorbed the cost and split it between our families. We continually reassessed what we *needed* to live on as opposed to what we *wanted* to live on. Many parents have been able to save money over the years. When the time came when they needed help, we found our parents wanted us to use their funds rather than incur costs on their behalf. My father has confirmed this fact, time and again by always wanting to pay his way.

When Dad was able to fly to Salt Lake City, and when I could make arrangements with a local surgeon to perform his surgery, expenses and pressures dropped dramatically. I could wait at the hospital while he was having surgery and after he was out of the recovery room and I was confident everything was fine, I returned to our home. I could visit Dad in the evenings at the hospital and spend my days at work. In Salt Lake City, because it was my home town, we all enjoyed support not only from family, friends and church; our work associates added another dimension of support. Upon his release from the hospital Dad was able to stay in our home until both he and I felt confident he could return to his home in Ohio. Expenses at our home were minimal compared to commuting back and forth from Salt Lake City to Ohio.

Whatever your situation—working couple, retired, single working adult, single parent—if you suddenly become responsible for the care of an elderly parent who is living in another city or state, your expenses can be reduced and your support system increased if you bring your parent into your home. While this option might be difficult even for a short duration, it may be your best option for reducing pressures as you meet this new responsibility. If, as in our case, there are two of you and you share the caregiving role, both your long distance and in-home caregiving will be easier. If you are a single working person, with or without children, and you attempt to keep your parent in your home, you may have no choice but to pool funds with your parents to hire someone for daytime care while you work. Some people may feel they have no choice but to place the parent in a nursing home. It's not an easy decision to make. If you try to care for a parent in your home, however, your ideas about what is and is not possible may change.

Keys to Caregiving

After our experience with Dad, we began to realize that sensible financial arrangements, clear communication with doctors and medical personnel, a firm grasp of the ins and outs of Medicare coverage and, perhaps most of all, maintaining a positive, optimistic attitude toward your parent are the keys to effective caregiving. As a caregiver, you will often face situations in which all four of these elements are important. Often it's hard to separate them from one another. For example, if you communicate well with your parent's doctor, your parent's medical problems will probably be kept under better control which will not only reduce the emotional toll on everyone but will reduce the financial burden as well. In fact, most people panic about money when they realize they're going to have to take care of an ailing parent. Talking with the doctor, understanding Medicare and being emotionally supportive do, ultimately, make it *cheaper* to take good care of a parent but it's always going to be more expensive to care for parents than to abandon them. Given this hard fact, it's best to face financial problems head on and come up with a realistic plan for coping with them.

Suppose, for instance, a parent in need of a great deal of care moves in with you. You and your significant other both work. You believe you need two incomes but one of you is going to have to quit. One option is for the person making the least money to stay home and then charge the parent for his or her care based on what the caregiver would have made on the job. If you decide to use this strategy, you must make a contract with your parent and report your salary from caregiving on your income taxes.

Of course, if you handle your parents' care on this basis, their savings may eventually run out. If your parent is receiving Social Security and maybe a small pension check, he or she could turn those funds over to you to help you cover expenses. Also, some of you may discover that a couple can adjust to one income while caring for a parent without added financial assistance. Sometimes, our sense of how much money we "need" has more to do with lifestyle than necessity.

If temporary nursing home placement is necessary, as it was for Dad, you must pay attention to the exact words the physician writes on his orders. For example, he may write "skilled nursing care" or "custodial care." We learned about what Medicare would and would not pay for the hard way. When the nursing home billed Medicare $3,000 for Dad's stay in the home, Medicare refused to pay the bill because the physician had not written orders for "skilled nursing care" even though Dad's placement had been medically necessary. Instead the doctor had inadvertently written his orders showing Dad needed only custodial care and at the time we didn't know the difference.

"Skilled nursing care" means the patient has had a recent medical setback and needs rehabilitation. "Custodial care" means the patient needs care for chronic problems and no medical emergency exists. For instance, if your parent cannot control urine or bowel movements and, therefore, requires more care than you are willing or able to give, the doctor's orders for nursing home placement would indicate only custodial care is needed. There is a financial difference between these types of care. Medicare will pay 100 percent of up to twenty days of skilled nursing care but will not cover custodial care.

Always check with the physician and with the hospital discharge planner prior to transferring someone to a nursing home to make sure the order has been written correctly, especially if skilled nursing care is required. After all, doctors are only human and, just like the rest of us, they make mistakes.

When a parent is being admitted into a Medicare-certified nursing home, there are three things you must ask your doctor and all three of these questions must be answered with a "yes" in order for the parent's stay to be covered 100 percent by Medicare for the first twenty days:

1. *Is admittance into the nursing home related to the patient's recent stay in the hospital?* If the answer is no, Medicare will not cover the charges because the hospital stay is a Medicare eligibility requirement.

2. *Has the patient been in the hospital three consecutive days prior to being admitted into a nursing care facility?* If the answer is no, the charges will not meet Medicare eligibility. On the first day in the hospital, if admittance is being done late in the afternoon, be sure to ask if it counts as one of the three days.

3. *Is the patient being admitted for skilled nursing care?* If the answer is no, Medicare will not cover the charges. Remember: Medicare will not cover charges for custodial care, only skilled nursing care.

When a person is discharged from the hospital and is to be admitted directly into a nursing home for skilled nursing care,

Medicare covers the cost only if the physician writes the orders showing skilled nursing care is necessary *and* care must be for the same condition that caused the person to be hospitalized. The facility should be Medicare-certified, the patient should be admitted within thirty days of a hospital admission and admission had to be for a minimum of three days.

We knew the last thing Dad wanted to do was pay a nursing home anything so, for motivational purposes, we told him Medicare would cover the first twenty days of his stay in the convalescent home at 100 percent after which there would be expenses for him to pay. His options were work hard and rehabilitate in twenty days or less and pay nothing, or stay longer than twenty days and pay his share. If he could get his strength back within those twenty days we felt we would definitely get him back to his own apartment.

Of course, we were not being *completely* honest with Dad concerning his stay in the home since we *did not* emphasize that Medicare would still be paying the lion's share of the bill beginning day twenty-one. Medicare Part A pays the full cost of covered services for the first twenty days of a Medicare benefit period. Starting on the twenty-first day, all covered services for the next eighty days are paid by Medicare, except for a daily coinsurance amount. In 1996, this amount was $92. Dad was responsible for paying the coinsurance. If he required more than 100 days, he would be responsible for all charges beginning with the 101st day because Medicare benefits run out after 100 days.

Emily and I knew when we gave Dad a twenty day deadline, we would reward his work by bringing him home within that period. We also were assessing his progress during that time, so that when he was released to go home, we would be more prepared to give him the care he would need. To show our love and support to him, we were always positive in everything we said and did. At no time did we speak negatively in Dad's presence about his situation or condition. By fulfilling our part of the commitment, we built trust and confidence with him. Set goals. Be positive. If you and your parent make a mutual commitment, keep your end of the bargain.

Nursing home costs can vary widely and depending on the area of the country, can easily exceed $50,000 a year. In Ohio, Dad had to pay $3,000 for his stay at the nursing home for thirty days. Although he was discharged after nineteen days, we had the nursing home hold Dad's room in case he had a problem and had to return to a nursing care situation. So he had to pay for those additional eleven days even though he didn't stay there. In addition to the charges Dad had for staying in the nursing home, he also was billed $500 for physical therapy. However, the Medicare *Explanation of Medical Benefits* notice (more about this form later) informed us Dad was not responsible for this portion of his bill because he had not been informed by the nursing home that Medicare would not pay for this service.

Caregivers will benefit from meeting financial needs, understanding Medicare and working toward better communication between themselves and their parents.

The Key to Obtaining Services: Your Physician

Emily and I were students in a two year Gerontology certificate program at the University of Utah during the time we were going back and forth from Salt Lake City to Ohio. An assignment in one of our gerontology classes required us to do an individual case study on one of our parents. We were to set up a support system consisting of community services, family, friends, neighbors and church. Since the two of us were providing long-distance caregiving for my father, I thought it would be a good idea for me to choose him as the focus of my assignment. Sharing this experience may be informative for other long-distance caregivers.

To comply with the class requirements, I had to call from our home in Salt Lake City to various agencies throughout

Ohio. It is not easy to find the many programs that are available for the elderly since they are listed under different titles and agency names. In 1991, the National Association of Area Agencies on Aging (NAAAA) established the *Eldercare Locator*, a toll-free 800 number for identifying the information and referral services provided by state government and Area Agencies on Aging throughout the United States. This service is part of the National Information and Referral Initiative implemented by the Administration on Aging in collaboration with NAAAA and the National Association of State Units on Aging.

Individuals calling the Eldercare Locator have access to more than 4,800 state and local information and referral service providers identified for every zip code in the country. The database also includes special purpose information and referral telephone numbers. Additional information about the National Information and Referral Initiative or the Eldercare Locator can be obtained by contacting the NAAAA. The World Wide Web address for the Eldercare Locator is http://www.aoa.dhhs.gov and the telephone number is 1-800-677-1116. This number is staffed from 9 a.m. to 11 p.m. (EST) Monday through Friday.

I was able to reach someone at the 800 number quite readily and they referred me to numerous agencies. The problem was not getting contact numbers; it was trying to reach people at these agencies. I experienced a great deal of difficulty trying to break through the many barriers that protected agencies from the people who were in need of their services. My efforts to contact Area Agencies on Aging (AAA) in the small, rural community of Wheelersburg, Ohio were, to say the least, frustrating.

Among the barriers to eligibility and limited services in small rural towns, I found trying to contact agencies that serve the elderly was expensive and time-consuming. I often spoke to people who were not properly informed about the services they offered and many times they would connect me to another agency that did not offer the service I was trying to find. I called some agencies at various times of the day and no one answered. As a result, I was not sure if the agency I was calling was the agency I wanted. Many of the agencies did not have an answering machine to leave a message and those that did never returned my calls. When I was able to locate an agency I was looking for, I discovered eligibility for programs was so diverse—based solely on income or solely on one's level of functionality—that qualifying was uncertain.

As an experiment, I tried to contact Aging Services in Salt Lake City. I found it equally difficult to get anywhere in my home town. When I was visiting in Wheelersburg, Ohio, I tried once again to telephone various Area Agencies on Aging to obtain services for Dad but encountered the same old runaround. In our experience, the key to obtaining the services needed is your physician. The best way to set up support through the system is to consult with the doctor who usually knows what services are locally available and what Medicare, Medicaid or other insurance programs will pay for.

A Balancing Act: Your Role in a Parent's Medical Decisions

Obviously medical care may be needed as people age and the body breaks down. If you are taking care of an elderly parent, you will probably have to make medical decisions on that person's behalf, when he or she is too sick to be consulted. Also, some elderly people are unaware of medical procedures that could make their lives much easier because they are poorly educated, afraid of doctors or just a bit behind the times. If your parent is unlikely to know his or her medical options, it's your job as caregiver to gather this information. Both these tasks, making medical decisions for an incapacitated parent and supplying information to an ill-informed one, requires objectivity. In the first case, you have to keep your *parent's* likely wishes rather than your own in mind. In the second case, you have to make sure you don't sway a weak elderly person toward your individual desire.

Emily and I had another lesson in how hard it is to take a role in guiding a parent's medical care on the morning of March 18, 1994, when we received another call from Dad's neighbor Nellie. She said Dad was back in the hospital. She had taken him to the doctor because he had not been feeling well and after a short examination, the doctor had Dad transported to the hospital by ambulance because he thought my father might have been having or might have already had a heart attack.

We immediately called Dad's physician, who informed us Dad was back in the hospital for congestive heart failure, accompanied by seventy percent kidney failure. The doctor had consulted with a cardiologist who believed Dad was in a life-or-death situation and suggested we might want to consider coming back to Ohio. He advised us of the urgency of placing a pacemaker in Dad's chest. The doctor wanted to know if we would approve the operation. Dad had previously said he wanted Byron and me to make medical decisions on his behalf because he couldn't understand medically what he was being told. We told the doctor to go ahead, knowing Dad held the opinion that if you can fix it, fix it. That afternoon the pacemaker was placed in his chest.

I called my brother and told him about the situation and informed him that Emily and I would be flying out the next day to be with Dad. We also told him we had discussed Dad's condition extensively and would be willing to bring him back to Salt Lake to live. Byron then released caregiving responsibility to Emily and me. He assured us of his support and requested we keep him informed. I told Byron to hang tight and we would contact him when we were with Dad.

It is extremely helpful and greatly appreciated if everyone supports the caregiver, especially those who do not want or are unable to share the primary responsibility themselves. That support can consist of contributing sound options or just saying thank you.

The next morning Emily and I were on the first plane out of Salt Lake City. When we arrived at the hospital we went directly to Dad's room and were pleasantly surprised to find him sitting up, talking with his cardiologist, apparently in a great mood. The doctor told us it was the pacemaker that had made the difference in Dad's recovery. Emily and I were pleased because we felt we had made the right decision when Byron and I approved having the pacemaker put in. My father was strong-willed, lucid and socially aware, had a great record for rebounding from physical adversity and was capable of getting around with little assistance. When we entered his room, his smile was a strong indication that he to was pleased with our decision.

While Dad's heart was now functioning well, thanks to the pacer, he still had difficulty dealing with a nagging urinary problem. During a conversation with my brother, Byron told me about a friend who has been using a supra pubic catheter for quite a few years. The man told Byron that having the catheter inserted supra publicly (above the pelvic bone in front) was the best thing he had ever done. The catheter allowed the urine to drain from the bladder to a bag attached to his leg. For convenience at night, a different kind of bag was used; both needed to be emptied when full. This freed him not only from pain but from the fear of embarrassing leakage.

We believed Dad could relate to Byron's friend because over the previous fifteen years, he had had to personally dilate or open his urethra (the canal through which urine passes) at least once a month so he would be able to urinate. Infection was always a major problem because Dad would not sterilize the instrument he used to perform this procedure, which is called a *sound*. Once dilated, he had to worry about uncontrollable leakage. After we discussed Byron's friend, Byron and I thought Dad might want to consider having a supra pubic catheter placed in his bladder so he would never again have to dilate himself. We decided to check with Dad's urologist to get his input about supra pubic catheters. The urologist agreed with the idea and felt Dad would be quite pleased with the catheter's placement. He informed us this was a very low risk procedure. We then suggested to Dad that he might want to consider having this procedure done. We gave him all of the information we had, then he decided for himself. When Dad was finally released from the hospital he brought two new things home with him: the pacemaker that had been implanted in his chest and a supra pubic catheter that had been placed in his bladder through a small hole in his abdomen.

When we first gave the go-ahead for a pacemaker, it was to save Dad's life; when we suggested he have a supra pubic catheter put in his abdomen, it was, hopefully, to give him a greater quality of life. Our only concern, when we gave the go-ahead for the pacemaker was that the device might keep his heart pumping even as other organs died and physical capabilities diminished. We were told the pacemaker would not prolong any sort of suffering for Dad because when other body parts quit functioning, the heart would just stop beating. Dad never questioned our decision to have the device implanted. When we asked him two years later about the pacemaker, he said "it may not be a great life and I'm not afraid of dying, but I don't want to die. The pacemaker has definitely made the difference." He also repeatedly expressed his pleasure with the catheter and our help in finding a solution to his urinary problem. His only regret was that he wished he had known about "this catheter" option years before.

Uprooting a Parent: The Humbling of Age

We dealt with a whole different set of reactions when moving Hardyn to Salt Lake than we had experienced moving

Lank to our home. We believe this was because Lank initiated the discussion on moving while we first broached the subject with Hardyn. Emily and I had numerous discussions about bringing Dad home to live with us in Salt Lake City and we both agreed it would be best for him if we did. There were many issues we had to cover to ensure we really knew what we were getting ourselves into. Since we knew it would not be easy to get Dad to agree to come live with us, we decided to move cautiously with our proposal.

To get things started, Emily and I went to Dad's senior citizen apartment complex to speak with the manager of the building. When we arrived, she told us she was concerned about Dad's age and worried he might not be able to live alone and care for himself. We shared her concerns and told her we would be talking to Dad later that day about what all three of us thought would be best for him and we would inform her of what we decided to do. We went back to the hospital to speak to Dad and told him about the conversation we had had with the apartment manager. We then invited him to come live with us in Salt Lake City. We were sensitive in acknowledging his feelings as well as showing him our excitement in having him live with us when he expressed his sadness about leaving his home and friends. The hardest part for us was expressing to him why we felt he could no longer live by himself and the actuality of what could or could not happen for him in Salt Lake City.

We reminded Dad that before he went to bed at night he needed to remove his catheter from the leg-bag that contained his urine and reconnect it to another collector called a down-bag; also, in the mornings he needed to reverse the process. He was not able to do either of these procedures without assistance. Neither was he able to clean his supra pubic catheter at the point where it entered into his body. This daily procedure is extremely important because it significantly reduces the possibility of infection.

In addition, when Dad was discharged from the hospital he was given a pacemaker kit. The pacemaker manufacturer would call him every third month to run a test to make sure the pacemaker was working properly. The kit included two bracelets that needed to be placed on his wrists and end-wires that needed to be connected to an impulse receiver so the manufacturer could hear the telephone test results. A magnet, a major part of the kit, needed to be placed on top of his pacemaker during transmission to the manufacturer. We pointed out that Dad would not be able to do any of these things by himself and if he stayed in his apartment he would have to have someone stay with him.

Finally, Dad had a wide assortment of medicines he needed to take. He often became confused about how much of each medicine to take and when to take it. A nitro-patch needed to be placed on his chest every morning and removed every evening. All of these things would need to be done at the right time and done properly or Dad would be in serious trouble.

I suggested we box up his belongings and get them ready for shipping to our home in Salt Lake City. He could bring anything he wanted within reason. I suggested selling furniture such as his couch, kitchen table, chairs and bed. We reminded him that our home was small and already furnished.

Another issue we knew we needed to discuss with regard to moving in with us was food. Our vacation experiences with Dad had revealed that when he was feeling good he never ate in his apartment. When he was feeling bad he would do the best he could within his home by fixing himself a bowl of soup or oatmeal. It was important to us that he understand our feelings concerning meals so eating would not become an issue later. Emily and I agreed that, to be fair, we needed to let him know our dietary habits are completely opposite from his. Inasmuch as we never eat at any particular time, seldom eat out and don't consume red meats or indulge in heavy meals, Dad could eat anytime he wanted, anywhere in the house. We would see he had the kind of foods he enjoyed eating, but he would more than likely be eating by himself most of the time. We knew Dad would have to make a major adjustment in this area.

Dad listened quietly. To have any chance of living in his own home, he would need someone there at all times, something he refused to do. He also ruled out moving to an assisted living facility. He decided we were his best option. So as much as he wanted to stay in his own place, he agreed to come.

When the elderly confine themselves to their home and do not take their medications, do not eat healthy foods, neglect personal hygiene, leave the stove on, walk without the assistance of a cane or walker when one is needed, they put themselves in danger. You may need to consider uprooting a parent when safety becomes an issue because of such self abusive behaviors.

When you initiate uprooting a parent, be gentle. Be prepared to explain what his or her new lifestyle will and will not include. Feelings and fears associated with a move suggested by the caregiver may be stronger than if the parent initiated the move. When you explain that your parent will have to live by someone else's schedule, expect resistance. Realize that living with now adult children under the children's ground rules is not what a parent really wants. Don't take negative reactions personally. Help your parent understand his or her options are few. Remember when we grow old, we too will have to live on someone else's schedule.

Recreating a Support System

We told Dad we hoped he understood that if he came out West to live with us we would all need to make concessions. There were many things we could do for him but we wanted to make it perfectly clear that we could only be *part* of a great support system. We could not be, nor did we want to be, his best friends who would pal around with him every day. When necessary we would take him where he needed to go but we could not be a taxi service; we could not drive him around the city on a daily basis just because he needed something to do. By explaining what he could expect from us, we established realistic boundaries. We also made it possible for Dad to value the new support system he would have and understand how it could make his daily life more enjoyable.

We reminded Dad that because he had lived in Salt Lake most of his life, many of his friends and relatives live only minutes away from our home and whenever he had been in Salt Lake City for a visit they had always come to see him. He would not lack friends or family contact. Lank, Emily's father, whom Dad had never met had been living with us in our basement apartment for four years. And then there was Hazel, my mom. Even though they had been divorced for years, my parents remained friends and on many occasions Dad, Mom, Byron and I had done things together. Mom would be someone Dad could visit in Salt Lake. We hoped they would also become good companions. Because we were asking Dad to come live with us, perhaps for the rest of his life, it was extremely important that he understood we loved him and wanted him but, as with any relationship, he also had to understand what he could expect from us.

We didn't know at the time if Medicare would classify Dad as homebound, but if they did not, he would have a number of programs to choose from. We could call Flextrans, a transportation service provided by the Utah Transit Authority for the handicapped and the elderly. Anyone who is unable to walk from home to the nearest bus stop is a candidate for this program. Flextrans would actually come to our home and drive Dad to a pre-selected location of his choice, then at a given time would return and bring him back home. There is a $.75 one way charge or $1.50 for a round trip. Most if not all states offer this kind of program for the elderly and the handicapped.

Anticipating he would say yes, Emily and I put Dad's name on the waiting list for a senior companion to come and visit him once every week for approximately four hours. As we mentioned earlier, senior companions are able-bodied seniors who volunteer to serve older people. If Dad wanted, his senior companion could take him to an occasional senior citizens' luncheon or to get his hair cut.

Additionally, our Salt Lake City Library offers a program called BOND (Books ON Delivery). Volunteers deliver books and books-on-cassette to homebound people. Books can be received in large print for those with poor eyesight. Also, where regular return time is twenty-eight days, for this program the return time is fifty-six days. This program provides a social outlet for the homebound person. Check with your community library for a similar program.

After we explained all of the challenges he was confronted with and after Dad heard our proposal, he said he was willing to give Salt Lake City a try. He made the decision to move to Salt Lake, in part, because he understood he needed the support team's assistance. When he accepted our invitation he was also acknowledging his understanding of what we would and would not do for him. We did reassure Dad that should his health fail, he could count on us to see he was properly and safely cared for.

When Dad's health declined, Emily and I did not have to shoulder the caregiving alone because his new Salt Lake physician set up an excellent support system. An aide came to our home three times a week to help him bathe. A physical therapist came to our home to assist him with strengthening and range-of-motion exercises. A nurse came every two weeks to monitor his vital signs, draw blood and take urine samples and replace the supra pubic catheter as needed. If all of these services are ordered by the doctor, they are covered by Medicare.

When needed, friends, relatives and church members provided us with a larger base of support in Salt Lake than Dad's friends and family in Ohio could have mustered.

Without this kind of support during declining health, it would only be a matter of time before Dad was back in the hospital or dead. Without the support system, Dad would have been totally dependent on himself and because of his lack of agility, forgetfulness, poor hand-eye coordination, sleeping habits and so on, he would not or could not do for himself what was necessary.

Medicare and the Homebound Impasse

To qualify for Medicare coverage for a home health service, you must meet four conditions.

1. You are confined to your home;
2. You require skilled nursing care, physical therapy or speech language pathology on an intermittent basis;
3. Your physician determines you need home care and sets up a plan with a home health agency to give you that care in your home; and
4. The home health agency is Medicare-certified.

When skilled nursing care is required for an injury or illness, Medicare will cover all charges if you use a home health agency and are confined to your home. You will not need to pay any deductible or be required to have a prior hospital stay. Medicare provides complete coverage for skilled nurses, home health aides, medical social workers and therapists for as long as the services are medically reasonable and necessary. Services cannot be provided full-time, only part-time or intermittently. Medicare will also cover the full cost of certain medical supplies, but only eighty percent of the approved amount for medical equipment such as hospital beds, oxygen supplies, walkers and wheelchairs.

If a certified Medicare home health agency is needed, ask your doctor or hospital discharge planners for assistance or look in the Yellow Pages of your telephone directory for one. Remember to work with your doctor and with Medicare to ensure you are Medicare covered.

While Medicare sees the classification "homebound" as an all or nothing classification, we see it in an entirely different light. Instead of assisting the elderly in getting out of the house, Medicare discourages it. Anyone can receive skilled nursing and therapy services if he or she is sixty-five or older and classified as homebound. Should a family member be in a position, however, to periodically take the person for a walk or even for a ride in the car, Medicare may determine the person is not eligible for services because he or she is able to leave the home, even though the person had to have help to do so.

It is our opinion that Medicare's policy discourages progressive improvement by not encouraging and supporting the individual or families that choose to bear the brunt of caregiving at home. When you place your elderly parent in a nursing home it's only a short time before Medicaid steps in to cover all of the cost of caregiving. If the government would support the caregivers and encourage positive living, everyone would win.

Closing Loose Ends and Moving On

When moving parents from their residence to yours, regardless of whether the move is from in-state or out-of-state, expect the move to be an emotional one for all concerned. For most people this would not be a joyous time. You are asking parents to leave old friends and routines behind, package limited belongings and move into your home. So allow them as much time as possible to make closures and, most importantly, encourage them to bring possessions that will keep their minds and bodies active. This will make their new life easier to adjust to. This was the approach we used for Dad.

Upon his release from the hospital, the three of us went back to Dad's apartment. Since his rent was due in four or five days, we decided to work quickly. To start, we took Dad to his bank where he closed checking and saving accounts. He also removed valuables from his safe deposit box and returned the keys. Next, we went to Dad's apartment so he could close his living quarters. We notified the manager of Dad's apartment complex we were taking Dad to Salt Lake City to live and he would not be returning. We also contacted relatives to tell them he wanted them to come to his apartment to say farewells. He wanted them to have whatever they wanted of his that he would not be taking with him. When relations arrived, closure was physically and emotionally disturbing and the only way Dad could cope with this situation was to leave his apartment and go visit his friend, Nellie, down the hall. He stayed with her until everyone had finally left and then returned to his quiet and now half-empty apartment.

Early the next morning we called Ohio Power and Light Co., the telephone and cable companies and other utility and service companies to have each service stopped and reroute the final bill to Salt Lake City. We spent the entire day packing what Dad had saved over the years and when we were through, we had eleven extra large shipping boxes. Several boxes were filled with pictures and old letters as well as things he had saved prior to retiring from the railroad, paraphernalia that included lanterns, locks, keys and various types of railroad pins. He had a coin collection and an old western gun — the last piece in a gun collection he had had for many years. These things, which were insignificant to us but important to him, were boxed and shipped to Salt Lake City. By having his things with him in Salt Lake City, he could continue to spend hours sifting through all of his different mementos, reminiscing about times long past.

One day when Dad was settled in our home, while I was sitting in the living room, he walked in holding a metal bar in his hands. He sat down and told me he had found it in Kentucky when he was with an old friend. He told me how looking at the metal bar brought back old memories. While sitting there, he just stared off into space, all the time stroking the metal bar. It was obvious to me that Dad was no longer in the living room with me; he was back, somewhere in time, with old memories of where he had been and who he had been with when he took possession of the metal bar. For the first time, I realized just how important the things he had saved over the years were to him, how they helped bring back memories of his past and keep his mind active.

Living Quarters Transitions and Financial Considerations

Emily and I knew we would be making adjustments to our living quarters when Dad moved in with us, but had not realized the extent to which we would have to change things. We also had not realized the expenses we would incur and the financial adjustment we would need to make. It didn't take long for us to find out what a difference sharing a home with Dad would make in our lives.

We continually reevaluated our living standards and looked at what was needed instead of what we wanted. It was important to us to make these adjustments so we could care for Dad, so he wouldn't have to walk this last part of his life with strangers. It was a way to show him we loved him. To start with, we moved from our large master bedroom to a smaller guest room so Dad would have as much space for his personal belongings as we could give him. At his request, we removed the bed from his room and replaced it with an electric hospital bed. We put a TV in his bedroom for his private enjoyment.

So Dad would not injure himself by tripping and falling, we removed our new sheepskin rug and coffee table from the living room. We removed everything of ours that could cause him to fall: carpets, throw rugs, cords. Eventually we had to strategically place chairs as we did with Lank throughout the house to help him maintain his balance so he could move unassisted from one room to another. We also removed from our living room a newly purchased, extra large, specially built recliner chair we had recently purchased for ourselves and replaced it with a motorized lift chair for Dad (styles and color coordination went out the window because we allowed Dad to choose his chair's color). We wired the living room and placed a telephone next to Dad's lift chair where it would be more accessible for him.

Since Lank was living in our basement apartment, Emily, Dad and I had to share one main floor bathroom. We installed grab bars so Dad could maintain his balance when getting in and out of the bathtub. To make it easier for him to get on and off of our low toilet, we purchased a potty chair with side bars on it (we eventually replaced the low toilet with a high handicap toilet and side bars). For easy access, we rehinged the bathroom door so it opened out.

Dad started spending much of his time during the daylight hours in his bedroom with the lights on—so much time, in fact, that he kept a small night stand lamp on practically twenty-four hours a day. He enjoyed time in his room rearranging belongings and going through old pictures, letters and other memorabilia. When Dad went to bed in the evenings, he slept with his light on. When I asked why, he said that if he woke up to use the toilet, he feared he would not find the light switch in time to light his way to the bathroom. Made sense to me.

Because we knew Dad had left his lights on all the time when he lived by himself , we accepted his habit of leaving his bedroom light on day and night. By saying nothing, we made it easier for him to adjust to his new home. Also, to counter his around-the-clock lighting, we purchased a light adapter with a guarantee that light bulbs would last thirty times longer than normal. We put one in each of his bedroom light fixtures, reducing the wattage approximately fifty percent. These devices, coupled with the two large windows in his bedroom, provided adequate lighting and saved on our electric bill.

Dad tended to sleep with his television on and the sound high. For this reason we did not want his television on once we were ready for bed. When we found him sleeping with the television on, we would simply slip quietly into his room and turn it off. If he was awake when we said good night, we programmed the television control's timing device so the TV would turn off thirty minutes after we left his room. Another option we presented Dad with was the use of ear phones connected to the TV but he showed no interest in them. As an alternative to late night TV, we sometimes suggested he play a favorite audiotape; he was generally agreeable. By the time the music was through playing he had fallen into a deep sleep.

Before Dad moved to Salt Lake City, he told us he would pay us $700 a month. We told him it wouldn't be necessary for him to pay anything, but we would appreciate it if he covered his own expenses and we in return would make sure he got whatever he needed. Each time the three of us discussed what we would do when we were in Salt Lake City, Dad would say, "I'm going to give you $700 a month." Then it was $600 a month. Then $500 a month.

When he first arrived in Salt Lake City, Dad gave us $500 a month to cover his expenses: food, incidentals and medicine. By the fifth month it was $500 every other month, then $500 every third month. By the eleventh month he had stopped giving us anything. Fortunately, we were able to absorb the additional costs. However, had we not been able to make ends meet, we would have had to ask Dad for help. The amount of hot water, laundry and bathroom supplies we went through in a week's time with Dad was amazing. Also, heat bills and grocery increased dramatically.

Our expenses increased while our income decreased. After three months, we determined Dad's care required one of us to adjust from full-time to part-time employment. Financially we were stretched and some months were tighter than others, but we were able to adjust our living standards without involving Dad in money issues because we scaled back our spending.

In-Home Caregiving Begins

When our fathers moved into our home we knew there would be small things we needed to do for them, small things to us, but big things to them: give physical support when they walked or dressed, assist getting in and out of a chair and in and out of clothes, button buttons, zipper sweaters, administer correct medicine at the right time. When they were incontinent, we cleaned the mess up, saying nothing. Oftentimes we offered such assistance and said nothing if doing so preserved dignity during a time when Lank or Hardyn found themselves unable to do something on their own.

The bathroom is perhaps the most dangerous room in a house for an elderly person. Since everything in the bathroom is made either of tile or metal, falls there are especially dangerous. For us to minimize the danger in our bathroom, we needed to make changes. Because of some problems Dad had early on, we could readily see what changes needed to be made and make them. All three of us had to learn to let go of what we used to think of as important and focus our energies on life and its many transitions.

When we took on the responsibility of caring for Dad we soon realized we would have to clean up after him and for him many, many times. Take for instance one night shortly after he first moved in. Dad woke up sick and went to the bathroom without asking for assistance. He had been in the bathroom about a half hour before he called for us. Startled, Emily and I jumped out of bed and hurried to the bathroom to see what was wrong. Through the closed door, he told us he needed our help but when we tried to open the door, we couldn't. We had not yet changed the bathroom door to open outward. At first we were only able to get the door open inward five or six inches but that was enough for us to see him laying on the floor with his body positioned against the door so we were unable to open it. Fortunately Emily was able to slip through the small opening and position Dad so we could open the door wide enough for me to fit through and once I was able to get into the bathroom we were able to give Dad the assistance he needed. When we got into the bathroom it was obvious Dad had been having bowel problems. There was fecal matter all over him, the toilet and floor.

We surmised later that when Dad had gone in to use the toilet, he no sooner had closed the bathroom door than his bowels started working. Instead of calling for us to come and clean up the mess, he had tried to clean it up himself, which had only exhausted him and made the situation worse.

Emily and I remembered my brother Byron telling us a similar situation had happened sometime back when he and his son, John, had been visiting Dad. Dad had gone to the bathroom and when he finished he had been too weak to get off of the toilet and had just sat there for about an hour. Byron checked on Dad periodically. The third time he went to the bathroom door, he called out asking Dad how he was doing. Dad said he needed help. When Byron tried to open the door, he also found Dad was lying on the floor between the toilet and the door, preventing Byron and his son from gaining entrance. The two of them worked for about an hour gently pushing the door, then getting Dad to inch back, before they were able to move Dad far enough away from the door so John, who was smaller than Byron, could get into the bathroom. Because of these two incidents, I removed our bathroom door's latch, hinges and striping and repositioned them so the door opens outward instead of inward, and I removed the lock on the door.

Now, if we needed to get into the bathroom fast because of a similar situation, we could.

We were told by someone in nursing services in Salt Lake that another "helpful" change we might consider would be to purchase a portable shower head with an extension hose because it would be much easier for Dad to use while being assisted with showering. Taking the advice of this professional, we purchased one of the best portable shower heads available. Dad had to hold onto the grab-bar with one hand to maintain his balance while standing in the bathtub, leaving him with one free hand to move the portable shower head around his body. And move it around he did. One morning as I was helping him with his shower, his concentration was on keeping his balance, not where he aimed the shower head. I got drenched; the bathroom got a soaking too. The next time I assisted him with showering I had him sit on the shower chair. Even though he was seated his attention was still directed toward keeping his balance. The bathroom and I got a second soaking. As far as I was concerned that was the end of Dad using a portable shower head. I replaced the portable shower head with a stationary one and found he could keep his balance and shower because the shower head could be pointed directly at him during the entire shower and he could use both hands to hold onto the grab bar rather than one.

If we had thought before we acted, we would have realized that because Dad had problems with standing and walking, he would not be a good candidate for a portable shower head with an extension hose. This experience taught me a valuable lesson: before buying any kind of device, evaluate both physical and cognitive abilities first.

Whose Autonomy is it?

Elderly people need to maintain a sense of autonomy, the feeling they can do things for themselves and have control over their own lives. While there may appear to be parallels between the behavior of an aged parent and a child, we must remember we are not caring for children. Our parent's have survived a lifetime of trials and losses, have already endured what the younger population has not yet had the opportunity to experience, and have shown themselves to be survivors. There is a delicate balance to caring for and helping elderly parents maintain some control over their lives. When taking on the caregiving role, stay away from parenting your parents. The time to take charge is when they are confused. The time to let go is when their controlling factors dictate they can understand the consequences.

Because we knew how important it was for Dad to maintain control over his life, we encouraged him to do as much for himself as he could whenever possible. Nevertheless, soon after Dad moved in, we discovered our encouragement and his lack of balance and cognitive processing placed us in a position where, when he exercised his right to do for himself, we experienced a lack of control over our time and daily schedule. His autonomy often interfered with our autonomy. For example, sometimes in the morning when Dad was alone in his bedroom, rather than waiting for one of us to come in and change the down-bag to his leg-bag, he attempted to do it himself, usually unsuccessfully, and did not realize the connection had not been completed correctly.

There were times when we found Dad walking around without his catheter connected to the down-bag or leg-bag or with the drain's valve left open and urine going down his leg, into his shoes, then onto the floor. One day we found him wearing his leg-bag upside down and he was unaware the urine was backing up on him. We tried to teach him how to do this procedure, but because of his weak hands and his inability to remember what we showed him, Emily and I felt his frustration on numerous occasions. After a number of these mornings, we started telling him we did not want him to change his bags because his getting urine all over his clothes, carpet and bedroom floor was creating more work for us. We told him the extra time needed to clean everything was causing us to change our work schedule too many times, that we could not afford to keep altering this schedule especially when we could avoid these situations if he allowed us to change his bags in the morning. Usually this resulted in a temporary change of behavior. But sooner or later he would attempt the task again and it always seemed to be on the morning of an important work day. Speak of Murphy's Law in action!

We tried various approaches to avoid these time consuming setbacks to our schedules. First thing in the morning we would put on Dad's leg-bag before he got out of bed (by moving quickly, we were able to keep him from changing the bag himself). Also, during the afternoons we started checking his leg-bag to determine if it needed emptying. If it did, we simply emptied it right away. We also checked on Dad regularly when he went to his bedroom. He would go to bed at anytime, day or night. So, we never knew for sure if he was going to bed or just going to his bedroom for privacy. We always asked, "Are you going to bed?" If he said "Yes" we would follow him, right then and there, into his bedroom and replace his leg-bag with his down-bag. If Emily or I had to get up during the night, we would peek into his room to check on him. If his bag was full, we drained it. When we learned to keep ahead of him this way, we "cut him off at the pass." Our caregiving became an easier task.

When Dad was feeling strong, he would challenge us and, we suspect, himself by saying he was going to walk to McDonalds by himself. Although I told him I did not think it was a good idea for him to walk the four blocks to McDonalds, I let him know it was his decision to make. I also knew, from his history on such walks, that if he got tired while he was out walking, he had no qualms asking complete strangers for a ride home. These strangers always were a positive experience for Dad.

So at ninety-one, when Dad embarked on these outings, he always reached his destination, one way or another. Yes, I experienced some anxiety when he took off like this, but not as much as Emily. I pointed out that it was his decision and as long as he was aware of the consequences and of where he lived and where he was going, I said, "go for it." I was okay with Dad's attempts to "go the distance." He survived and enjoyed meeting the challenge he set for himself. But Emily's days were usually consumed with worry as she tried to balance Dad's need for confirmation that he could still do something by himself and her anxieties toward an elderly parent out walking alone, subject to the dangers of falling, having someone take advantage of him or becoming exhausted and disoriented.

No Marathon Runner: Living with a Parent's Physical Limitations

We knew Dad, at ninety-one, would never again move, react or think as fast as he once did, regardless of what he did. While it only took us a few seconds to walk thirty feet, it took him nearly ten minutes to walk the same distance and, on occasion, because he moved so slowly, sometimes he forgot where he was going and why. There was one time when Dad and I were sitting in the living room and he told me he needed to use the toilet and pronto. We stood up, he gathered his balance and we started toward the bathroom. Suddenly he stopped and then he turned toward a TV tray that stood next to his chair and started gathering up some of his things to carry into his bedroom. When I finally got him started in the right direction he stopped once again, stooped over and tried to pick up his shoes from the floor. It made us very nervous when he bent over to pick something up from the floor because he could easily lose his balance and fall. I told him to leave whatever he wanted and I would bring it to him after he was through in the bathroom. As we entered the hallway leading into the bathroom Dad suddenly turned to go into his bedroom. He had forgotten that we were hurrying to get him to the toilet. I had to remind him where he wanted to go.

Because he had little control over his bowels, it was important for him to get the quickest jump possible on going to the bathroom when he felt the urge coming on. On a number of occasions, because he moved so slowly, he was unable to get to the toilet before his bowels started working and he defecated in his shorts and on the bedroom or bathroom floor. This was embarrassing and frustrating for him but even though he was concerned about his bowel problems, it did not seem to discourage him from eating the foods that made the problems worse. We tried to get him to eat foods with more bulk and fiber in them. We also tried to get him to drink at least eight glasses of water each day. One of those glasses of water contained a heaping tablespoon of orange-flavored Natural Vegetable Powder for regularity. At first, getting him to drink the powdered glass of water was like trying to pull teeth out of a sick grizzly bear, but after a while he saw how it helped control his watery bowel movements and was more willing to drink it.

In a three year period, Dad went from a large, 220 pound man to a small, 136 pound man. His frail, skinny legs were barely able to carry his weight, let alone allow him to walk as he used to. We have no doubt he became frustrated with himself as well as with us because he had no control over these physical functions. There were times we became equally frustrated with how we should handle certain situations. But we were never frustrated about something over which Dad had no control like being incontinent or slow. Showing impatience at these times would only create more anxiety for a frail old man already having to cope with a number of limitations.

It is important to remember that as our bodies age we slow down. We do not move or think as fast as we once could and our reaction time is not as quick as it used to be when we were younger. While caring for an elderly person, do not get upset when you're trying to get him or her to do something. Instead, recognize that person's age and limitations. Your challenge will be to get off the fast track, to patiently slow down and look for solutions to the problem at hand. Slowing down may be frustrating for you, but think how frustrating it must be for elderly people to try to walk across the street at a crosswalk when no one stops to let them cross or when they are at a busy intersection and the light changes before they can make it across the street because the timing is set for younger, more limber bodies. As our population ages, it is apparent we will all need to change gears eventually.

Chairs with Wheels

When the legs start to give out, chairs with wheels can be a great asset in a variety of situations. One area in particular where we needed a chair with wheels was at the dinner table. Dad had difficulty moving his chair away from the table because of the soft carpet, so we had him move to a sturdy swivel chair with arm rest and wheels that sat comfortably under the table. When Dad was through eating, he merely turned to his right, stood and then walked with his walker to his lift chair.

One day the three of us were discussing wheelchairs, because of Dad's slowness. We all agreed that it would be a good idea if he had one. Emily and I thought it would be great because of the time it would save us whenever we took Dad to the doctor. Instead of walking he could ride. Dad's slowness had been the number one complaint of friends and relatives who took him places. It took a long time for him to just get out of his chair, let alone walk anywhere. Dad wanted the wheelchair because he thought he could just get in it and take off, something he soon realized was not possible. I looked in the classified section of the local newspaper under Medical Equipment for Sale. I found a wheelchair for sale and made an appointment for Emily and me to look at it. When we arrived at the seller's residence we were pleasantly surprised when we saw the wheelchair. It was practically new in appearance and the owner only wanted $100 for it. New, the wheelchair would have sold for $450 to $500. We bought it. When we arrived home, I told Dad we had purchased a wheelchair that was in great shape and surprisingly he responded by saying he did not want one. But since *we* wanted it, we kept it.

When Dad first saw the chair, he had nothing good or bad to say about it and for the following four or five days we had no real opportunity to use it. Around 4:30 one afternoon, however, when Dad, as usual, had been inside for the entire day, I asked him if he would like to catch a breath of fresh air. I explained to him I could take him around the block in the wheelchair. He said that would be fine. I told him I would put the chair in the front yard and when he was ready, I would help him outside. He continued to just sit in his lift chair and for five minutes or longer he continued to play with his watch chain. I told him if we were going to go we needed to go then or I would not be able to go at all. Again I asked him if he still wanted to go and he said yes. Then he asked, "Would you like to go to the Big M?" (Dad's name for McDonalds) I told him I had time to take him around the block in his wheelchair and would be happy to do that because he could get out of the house and get some fresh air, but Big M was out of the question. I said Emily would be home from work shortly and I wanted to be home when she arrived.

Dad said it did not matter, meaning forget about going around the block. He did not make any movement to get up so rather than coax him, I walked outside, picked up the wheelchair and brought it back into the house. I went back to my office feeling frustrated with him for not being appreciative of what I was offering to do. I'm sure he also was frustrated about being limited in what he could do but I had no tolerance that day for playing any games with him, so I went back to my business. That evening no one mentioned the chair and Dad was back to his talkative self. He did not use his wheelchair too often but there were times when we had to use it just to get him from one room to another.

For someone who has a parent who is not as limited as our Dad but is still slow in moving around, a wheelchair can add to their enjoyment in such places as flea markets and museums. These activities are usually held in large facilities and cover long distances. When using a wheelchair for browsing through these places, all of your parent's energy and all of your patience will not be worn out.

If Dad had to be at a certain location at a certain time, such as the doctor's office, it was a must that we start to get him ready well before his appointment. If we needed to leave the house by 11:30 a.m., we had him start getting ready somewhere around 9:30. If we were not prepared for Dad's slowness it was very frustrating to try to get him anywhere on time. Knowing how he felt at a particular time of day was also important. If he did not feel strong in the legs and his balance was poor, we had him use his walker rather than his quad cane because it was more stable. We tried to have him walk as much as possible but if it became necessary, we used his wheelchair.

We knew Dad would be slow but if we took a few moments to assess his physical condition on the day of his appointment, we could figure out how much assistance he needed to get ready and decide whether he should use a cane, walker or wheelchair. The secret was planning ahead.

Tell-Tale Signs: Identifying Urgent Situations

There are many tell-tale signs we look for in our everyday life that alert us to potential problems. These signs come from many directions. Whether it be the color of body fluids, emotional outbursts, the use of specific words or an urgent tone of voice, we are continually looking for indicators that will help us determine the importance of what is taking place. For instance, Emily and I have never had a problem in the morning sharing our one small bathroom. If either of us has to be out of the house at a certain time, we merely give priority to the person needing to leave first. Because of Dad's weak bowel problem, however, we had to give him priority: when he had to go, he had to go. We learned that when he knocked on the bathroom door when one of us was trying to get ready for work, we needed to pay attention to what he said. If he asked, "Are you in there?" or, "How long are you going to be in there?" or, "Are you going to be out soon?" we did not just run out and let him in. We asked him *specific questions* such as, "Do you have to sit on the toilet?" We never asked, "Do you need to use the bathroom?" Of course he needed to use it; that's why he was asking us how long we would be. We questioned him further because after living by himself for so long and having the run of his own home, he had not had to be concerned with the needs of others. There were times when we left the bathroom at his request and once he was in the bathroom he had forgotten that we needed to get back in. He would clean his false teeth, comb his hair, wash, shave or do any number of other things, totally disregarding our needs.

Expressions we listened for and responded to immediately included, "Are you going to be much longer?" or "I need to get in there," or "I have to go," or "I need to use." These urgent remarks signaled us to move out fast and help him out of his clothes and get him seated to expedite his time in the bathroom. Once we were out of the bathroom and he was on the stool we reminded him that on completion he was to inform us so we could help him out.

These are the trials of sharing one small bathroom. At first we had problems sharing the bathroom with Dad because we were not able to read his signs. Once we understood what he was really trying to say, we were able to cope with having three people using the same bathroom. It is important to listen carefully to what is actually being said.

When relaying information to Dad's doctor or home nurse, there were three things we found to be very helpful in identifying a possible problem: a thermometer to take Dad's temperature, a stethoscope to monitor his vital signs and "knowing our colors." We learned the importance of noticing the color change of any sputum, fecal matter or urine he expelled.

Sometimes when Dad was not feeling well, his lungs became congested because of fluid build-up. When we talked on the telephone with Dad's nurse or doctor, we informed them of the color and consistency of sputum. This gave them a better insight of what the problem may have been and how best to treat it. For example, if sputum's color is rusty, brown, bloody or green, there is a higher possibility that a bacterial infection such as pneumonia, bronchitis or tuberculosis is developing. The color yellow is often associated with heavy smokers and viral infections. Be careful not to confuse the color of the sputum with food or drinks that have been recently consumed. Any of these colors with or without a fever made us suspicious. Older people do not always respond to an infection with an elevated temperature. They may be seriously ill and have minimal elevation of temperature.

We also checked the color of Dad's stools because certain colors indicate potential problems. For example, brown, tan and green stools are generally considered normal. Abnormal colors — clay, black and tarry — can, unless the person is taking iron supplements, indicate liver disorders, hepatitis, GI bleeds or cancer. Blood in the stools can indicate cancer, diverticulitis, colitis or hemorrhoids.

Finally, we looked for signs of blood in Dad's urine. If the color was rusty looking, there was probably blood present. If it was clear and contained floating particles, it was possible that a urinary tract infection was developing. If there was blood present anywhere we reported it immediately to his nurse or doctor. Do not try to diagnose a parent using this list! Just remember that noticing the color of sputum, stools and urine, then relaying this information to the nurse or doctor can help them make decisions on how to treat the patient.

A strong display of emotions is another tell-tale sign, and can indicate a potential physical problem. Emily and I found that when everything became a big issue with Dad, when he complained of being cold, was easily upset and confused, he was developing a urinary tract infection.

Over the years I'm sure Dad had taken various antibiotics inappropriately which is probably one of the reasons that later in life he had infections that were resistant to many antibiotics. People have written numerous articles on antibiotics and how many bacteria are becoming impervious to medicine. A common form of staphylococcus which causes everything from pneumonia to wound infections is now resistant to all antibiotics except Vancomycin which is considered the drug of last resort.

Because of Dad's resistance to so many antibiotics, his urinary tract infections usually did not clear up until the infection got so bad he was downright sick and bedridden. By noting certain signs we were prepared for what was to come. Once Dad was bedridden, the doctor would have him admitted to the hospital where he could be put on powerful intravenous antibiotics which act faster and more effective than those taken orally.

Remember first and foremost, you are family. Sometimes things get tough but you have to be able to work through the trying times by attempting to understand what is causing or has caused the problem. Difficult? Yes. Can it be done? Yes. Alone? No!

Emily, and I chose to work through trying situations rather than release our loved one to the care of casual acquaintances within a nursing home. The challenge to us, while we were caring for our father, was in helping him maintain his dignity. We discovered that when we identified the tell-tale signs of an on-coming medical problem, Dad responded positively when we proceeded with light conversation or silence as we slowly, gently went about doing things for him.

Purchasing Medication

Only the newest antibiotics were effective for Dad and they cost an arm and a leg. Most of the antibiotics he took cost between $3 and $6 per pill. Other regularly prescribed medications were also expensive but thanks to some friendly advice from an aide who bathed Dad three times a week, we were able to purchase some expensive medications from the home health company in our state at prices well below the prices we had paid at a large, supermarket pharmacy.

I gathered all of Dad's medication and the cost for each item before calling the Professional Nursing Service's (PNS) home health pharmacy. They could beat most prices. For example, I could purchase sixty cimetidine 400 mg tablets for $25.45 from PNS pharmacy. We were paying $41.60 for the same drug at the pharmacy in a large grocery store chain. Thirty units of Nitro-dur 0.1 mg/hour patch cost $42.20 at the supermarket pharmacy. The cost at PNS was $27.20. We could not purchase all of Dad's medication at PNS at a savings, but the price difference was always less than a dollar on those specific items PNS could not beat.

One thing PNS pharmacy does that really impressed me was that when they fill a prescription for a name brand pharmaceutical, they provide a computer printout of any available generic product. If every pharmacy was to do this, there could be a tremendous savings on prescriptions for all people, not just the elderly. The grocery store pharmacy claimed it would meet anyone's price, but when the pharmacist saw the PNS price, he said he could not honor his pharmacy commitment. This is because PNS buys on a contract that is not available to the grocery chain.

I called the PNS pharmacist and asked him how his pharmacy was able to outsell a large chain store. I learned PNS Pharmacy is a statewide, non-profit organization dedicated to providing the highest quality IV therapy, oral medications and nutritional support services in the patients' home. PNS has hospital purchasing power because it is a closed-door pharmacy, which means that not just anyone can walk in and purchase medication. Only PNS patients can use the PNS pharmacy.

It is possible there are other programs like PNS with similar services for their patients. We encourage you to investigate whether any home health agencies offer such services in your area. If you find a program similar to PNS, compare costs to what you are paying and you could be pleasantly surprised. Maybe you will even want to change nursing services.

Home Health Care Providers

As we had speculated, the time came when Dad's physician was able to set him up with a home health nurse, aide and therapist. Dad's nurse came to the house once every two weeks to check his progress and once a month to change his supra pubic catheter. An extremely competent aide visited Dad every Monday, Wednesday and Friday to check his weight, vital signs and give him a bath plus assist him in dressing. This gave all of us a break; it gave Dad some privacy. About the time Dad finished his bath on Monday, in came his senior companion, also a very competent individual. With the two services combined, Emily and I had approximately five to six hours of "free" time to run errands and take care of personal business. We were very appreciative of these services.

On the other hand, other services were unappreciated. Specifically, one physical therapist who came into our home was very disappointing. In our opinion, she did little to help Dad achieve the recovery goals set by his doctor. When a physician sets goals for a patient with poor circulation, balance or a falling problem, it is the therapist's responsibility to see those goals are achieved. Normally, goals for a patient with a falling problem include but are not limited to independent transfer of patient from chair or bed, standing and walking, increasing strength, mobility and being able to get up from the floor after falling. Also, the doctor would have the home surveyed and modified for safety measures.

When Dad's therapist came to our home to aid him with a falling problem, she was suppose to work with him fifteen to thirty minutes three times a week. However, the first thing she did was make several calls to her next appointments, informing them of her planned departure and possible arrival times. Then she would call her company, noting where she was and what changes she anticipated in her schedule. It is our understanding that Medicare paid approximately $130 to $140 an hour for these services.

A flaw in the Medicare system? We observed more times than not that our elderly parents did not get what the therapists were paid to provide. One therapist told us she was semi-retired and my Dad was her only client. She appeared to be between sixty-five and seventy years old and she could not have weighed more than 100 pounds soaking wet. Since we had no confidence in her ability to move Dad up or down the stairs, we didn't want her to take him for walks outside because if he had lost his balance on the cement steps, we didn't think she could prevent him from falling. After the first six weeks, however, we knew we needn't to worry about her taking Dad for a walk because she never tried to get him up for more than a few steps. She stood before Dad while he was seated and had him raise his hands above his head. She had him do one, sometimes two sets of ten, raising and lowering his arms. She would do the same amount of sets having him raise and lower his legs while sitting. It became apparent that the exercises she was having him do, while good for his circulation and getting the kinks out, were in no way helping him with his problem of balance. Dad was capable of doing much more. Her total time spent with him was something like ten to fifteen minutes and this included her phone calls. We discontinued her services.

Another distressing situation we experienced was when Dad was walking toward the bedroom door and, with his down bag still attached to the bed, he pulled the supra pubic catheter from his abdomen. I reported this incident to our home health nurse and she had a substitute nurse call me. She asked what size catheter Dad needed and I suggested she bring both a twenty and a twenty-two gauge supra pubic catheter in case the twenty-two was too large. Since Dad had been living with us, he had had six or seven different nurses put a dozen or more supra pubic catheters in his abdomen, and occasionally, when asked, I assisted them. On this particular Saturday evening, I offered my assistance and it was rejected outright.

It can be painful when a large gauge catheter is placed in the abdomen, especially if probing and moving it about is necessary to get it positioned correctly. While I was in my home office, I heard the nurse talking to Dad about placing the catheter in its proper position. Because Dad was experiencing considerable pain, I asked if I could assist her. She again said no. Later on, I heard her say to Dad that she finally had the catheter in place, but was not certain why urine was not passing through. She suggested that perhaps Dad needed to drink more water and since she needed to leave, she would telephone me in one hour to see if any urine was in Dad's bag. When she called, I felt Dad's bag through his slacks and it was still empty. The nurse said she would return, remove the catheter and try again.

She was nervous when she arrived, and began by explaining that her supervisor never mentioned supra pubic catheters were needed. She assumed they were "foley" catheters, used to drain urine from the *penis* and that's where she had placed it. His penis had not been open for years. I was mad as hell because she had put Dad through such unnecessary pain and discomfort for days to follow. She made what I thought was an enormous mistake and she knew it. In our earlier conversation, I was certain that when we discussed gauges, I mentioned the supra pubic catheter by name.

I was not only upset with the nurse, but with myself. I kept thinking, this would not have happened if I had been with Dad. I ignored one of our major rules: stay visible.

Since this incident happened on a Saturday, I called Dad's urologist Monday to ask if the nurse may have done any long-term damage. He assured me she had not and everything would be all right. By Tuesday, Dad was no longer hurting and the doctor said he would be fine.

The nurse knew she made a mistake and she was apologetic. I could see the hurt in her face. She called over the weekend to check on Dad and apologized continually. I told her not to worry and assured her we needed to move forward and not dwell on the past.

The services that are available to the elderly are extremely beneficial—when the providers perform them properly but disturbing when they do not give 100 percent. In spite of our experiences with the physical therapists and on-call nurse, we believe strongly in the home health program over the alternative of long-term nursing home care. For the most part the service providers who assisted Dad were wonderful, caring, professional people whom we respected and in whom we had extreme confidence. They were also people who treated us as part of the caring team.

VALIDATION

In 1995, Emily and I attended a meeting at a local care center where a facilitator lectured about a technique called *validation*. In addition to her lecture, we watched a video and were given an information sheet demonstrating how to do validation. The care center showed us plenty of evidence that validation therapy works. It is a tested model of practice that helps old, disoriented people reduce stress and enhance dignity and happiness.

Validation was developed between 1963 and 1980 by Naomi Feil. This therapy accepts an old person's return to the past. As Feil said in her videotape,

> In old age, people can survive through hindsight. When eyes fail, they see with the mind's eye. When hearing fails, they hear sounds from the past. They see childhood scenes when recent memory and friends die. They restore the past to relive good times and resolve the bad in this final struggle to find peace.[1]

Validation helps the elderly win. One evening I was helping Dad prepare for bed, when he said he was going to go back to Ohio to see his old friend Herb (Herb managed the bank where Dad had once done business). Dad said he wanted to put some things into and take some things out of his safe deposit box. I responded, "You don't have your safe deposit box anymore, you . . . . " He cut me off with, "I do have it." To which I responded, "No. You closed out your savings and checking accounts along with your safe deposit box and you brought everything you had to Salt Lake City. Your coin col-

Feil, Edward. (Producer & Director). (1988). Validation therapy [Videotape]. Cleveland, OH: Feils Products.

lection is in the bottom drawer of your dresser over in the corner of your bedroom. . . . " He suddenly got angry and said, "You know everything. I still have my safe deposit box back in Ohio and I don't see why you're trying to pick a fight with me."

Dad was so angry, I knew I had to do something to calm him down and fast, so I said, "Dad, now that I think about it, you may be right, you may still have your safe deposit box." I asked him if he remembered when he was at the bank the last time and he said, "No." I asked him if he knew who had the key to his box and he said he did. Then I asked him where he had put it and he told me he could not remember. I told him I would help him look for his key in the morning and what he could do to help me find it. I told him not to worry, that I would help him find his key so when he was back in Ohio he would have no problem getting into his safe deposit box. He smiled and said, "Good old Herb, he really is a nice guy!" Within moments Dad was completely at ease. I had validated his mind's eye visit to a time long past. He was smiling and reminiscing about the good old days and how he and Herb had such good times together. Dad never again brought up the subject of his safe deposit box.

We found it equally important for Dad's morale to validate his goals. Six months after he moved in with us, he started making plans for his return to Kentucky. He wanted to see and visit everyone he knew. Our relatives said there was no way he could go back and still take care of himself and they let him know what they thought. On the other hand, Emily and I constantly told Dad he could do it and we would work with him to see that he would. We didn't really think Dad would be able to make the trip but he was determined to go back and, because he had set a goal for himself, we supported him 100 percent. We did not realize he wanted to be in Kentucky on Memorial Day so he could put flowers on his mother's and father's graves (he is buried next to them). As we got closer to

Memorial Day weekend, we could see he was truly determined to go.

While making plans for Dad's trip to Kentucky, and within a few hours of being admitted to the hospital for a falling and incontinent problem, Lank suffered a massive heart attack. Dad took the news with little emotion: he had been living with us for one year but neither Dad nor Lank had made a real effort to get to know each other. Dad asked about the seriousness of Lank's condition. I replied Lank probably wouldn't be with us much longer. Then Dad asked what we would do with Lank's body. I told him Lank had a pre-paid burial agreement similar to his, that he wanted to be buried with his wife in Harrisburg, Pennsylvania and that we would see his wishes fulfilled.

On May 15, 1995, Lank died. When we gave the news to Dad, he said, "Poor Lank. He was a nice guy." Six days later, Emily and I returned from Lank's burial. I began making final plans for Dad's trip to Kentucky.

Dad wanted to spend one month in Kentucky and we knew there was no way he could do that and not have major problems. We told him one week would be the longest period of time he could safely spend there and he agreed he would only stay one week. Since it was our intention to do whatever we could to make his wish a reality, we contacted my brother Byron and told him Dad was going to Kentucky, and he wanted to be there for Memorial Day so he could put flowers on his parents' graves. We asked Byron if he could go back and stay with Dad at our Aunt Ruby's farm and see he got around safely. We were willing to write directions about what medicine Dad needed and when. Byron also needed to know about proper catheter and urine bag care.

Although traffic would be terrible over Memorial Day weekend, Byron agreed to drive the 1,500 miles to our Aunt Ruby's home. He said he would see to it that Dad was able to go and do whatever he wanted. Later, Byron called to let us know he could only take off four of the six days Dad was planning to be in Kentucky which meant Byron would leave two days before Dad was ready to return to Salt Lake and Dad's 83-year-old sister would have to provide care by herself. Our biggest concern was how Byron and Aunt Ruby would deal with Dad's supra pubic catheter. We were not sure they would be able to follow our directions regarding his catheter's because they had no training. Infection was our major concern, but we believed the extra two days with Aunt Ruby could result in only minor problems that we could correct once he was back with us in Salt Lake City and that turned out to be just the case.

Because of the time difference between the East Coast and the West and because it was better for Dad to skip medication instead of take it too soon or too late, Aunt Ruby was instructed to discontinue Dad's medicine the morning of his departure, so we could put him back on schedule when he returned. The first thing we did when he arrived home was check his catheter to see if it needed cleaning. It looked pretty good but we cleaned it again just to be sure.

The bottom line was Dad proved everyone wrong. He set a goal for himself and he was able to reach that goal with our support. Dad would have gone to Kentucky regardless of what anyone said so it was important for Emily and me to set up a support system with members of our family to make his trip possible. If we had not arranged a support system, things probably would have turned out poorly.

About a year after Dad arrived in Salt Lake City, his attention turned toward another goal: getting around the city by himself. For safety reasons, he had reluctantly given up driving. Because he felt he could still control some type of vehicle, he told us he would like to get a three-wheeled bicycle which, hopefully, would help him regain some lost independence. "I could ride the three-wheeler to the store, the Big M, or to visit friends," he said. Once again, everyone tried to talk him out of buying a bicycle; each person had his or her own reason why Dad should not ride it. To Emily and me, it was not important whether he could ride it or not, what was important was for us to validate his interest in finding a three-wheeled bicycle.

We well knew Dad could not ride a three-wheeled bicycle but helping him research his interest brightened his days. The three of us started looking in the classified ads to see if anyone had one for sale. We also checked with bicycle shops and found out three-wheelers were not popular. Finally, we found one for sale for $300. Emily and I drove to the address given to us and there was an old three-wheeler sitting in the front yard. We approached a woman who was standing next to the bicycle and inquired about the possibility of taking the bicycle for our 91-year-old father to see. After hearing our story the woman agreed to let us show it to Dad. He thought it was too old, that it needed new tires and a paint job and was too expensive. We returned it and he never mentioned wanting a bicycle again. By searching for the three-wheeler, we validated Dad's dream. The rest was up to him and Dad finally decided the dream was not for him.

Naomi Feil says the key to validation is accepting the time-frame chosen by the speaker. Use nonthreatening, factual words: talk about who, what, where, when, how. Avoid asking why, because it makes the speaker justify his or her responses. Ask about long ago: a disoriented elder will enjoy telling stories about long ago. Also it will help reduce stress and enhance dignity and happiness.

The "Big M" Blackmail and a Dose of "Reality Orientation"

Sometimes a dose of "reality orientation" is the only way to get across an important message to your parent. Unlike validation, where you try to relate to a senior's realm of reality, reality orientation brings the elderly into the present and attempts to remind them how things are now. Emotionally, it is hard to do reality orientation but if it works, a noticeable change for the good will be seen.

In spite of what we told Dad about our eating habits before he moved in, meal time still became an issue we had to confront. Dad had a tendency to retain fluids. This caused his feet to swell which made it more difficult to walk. His doctor suggested a salt-free diet would reduce his foot problems. In spite of this, he didn't want to give up salt any more than he wanted to avoid the foods that caused his watery bowel problems. I asked Dad's doctor if it would be OK if Dad had his favorite meal, McDonalds' sausage and biscuit. There is a lot of salt in sausage but at Dad's age, he wanted to eat what he liked, not what we told him was best for him. As he said so many times, "What's it going to do, kill me?" The doctor had no problem with him having his sausage and biscuits maybe twice a week, but told us not to make it part of his daily diet.

Because Dad wanted to eat what he enjoyed, we tried to figure out ways he could do so and still maintain ambulatory control. Sandwiches from the Big M helped conjure good memories of meeting and conversing with old acquaintances. It reminded him of stories which he then shared with us, his nurse, aide and senior companion. So two days a week we saw he got his McDonalds treat.

Once, when no one had come to visit Dad during a particular week, I gave in and drove him three consecutive days to McDonalds for a sausage and biscuit breakfast. The next morning, Dad came into the living room and said, "Do you want to drive to the Big M to get breakfast. I'll treat." We told him not today, explained that Emily and I had already eaten and reminded him he had already eaten more biscuits and sausage the last few days than his doctor wanted him to have in one week. He didn't like this response and his reaction caused our feelings to escalate from empathy to irritation. He pouted most of the morning and refused to eat what Emily prepared. Dad's refusal to eat anything except food from the Big

M was his form of blackmail. Traveling regularly to the Big M pleased Dad, but it was time consuming for us.

On this particular morning, in front of Dad I said to Emily, "Did you know that Dad doesn't believe we do enough for him? He refuses to eat because we won't run to the Big M for his breakfast. He's probably right, we do not do anything for him. We only make sure he gets his 7 a.m. medicine, change his catheter from the down-bag to the leg-bag, put a new nitro patch on his chest, assist him in dressing and wash his dirty shorts and clothing. We clean him up when he gets sick, as he often does, regurgitating during the night and many times we have had to give him a suppository to control the sickness. We make sure he has his 3 p.m. medicine and his 11 p.m. medicine. At 11 p.m., we take off his leg-bag and empty it of urine and then we clean it and put his down-bag on for the night. We remove his nitro patch and we clean the opening to his abdomen where the supra pubic catheter enters his body. So I can understand why he does not feel we do enough for him." Dad did not say a word but his demeanor showed that what I said registered.

For some time thereafter Dad ate the meals we prepared at home and on occasion, he actually expressed his appreciation for what we did. I never felt good about the way I reacted to Dad's blackmail even though it produced the results I wanted. We knew we had to come up with a way for Dad to understand the reality of our situation without destroying his dignity. After many hours of discussion, Emily and I decided to simply remind him that we did not have the time, money or the luxury of being retired to run to the Big M every morning to purchase his breakfast. This response was well received by Dad when he asked us if we wanted to go somewhere that would cost us money and take time during busy work days. Having worked hard and for as many years as he did, he could relate to both responses.

Be careful with reality orientation because it can result in good or poor reorientation. Poor but effective reality orientation changes your parent's behavior but damages his or her dignity. Be careful to always communicate in a caring way. You can hope to develop better communications with elderly parents if you are sensitive but it can be a struggle at times.

Not Acknowledging the Caregiver

Giving long-term care to a parent who is not willing to acknowledge what is being done for him or her can become frustrating. Emily and I had our moments of frustration with Dad. One morning when I asked Dad if he would like something from the Big M, he said yes, so I drove to McDonalds and purchased a biscuit and sausage for him. When I returned, he asked if there was a hardware store close by where he could get something he needed. I told him there was but I did not have time to drive there then. I suggested that perhaps I could pick up what he needed the following day. Unexpectedly, he responded, "I didn't ask you to go anywhere for me and I never have." He also pointed out that he has never asked for anything from Emily and me. Technically, he was right: he had implied he wanted certain things done and we had volunteered to do them, but he has never actually asked us to do anything for him. Nevertheless, an undercurrent of quietness filled the house for most of the day. Dad felt trapped and we felt he had dismissed everything we had done for him.

The next morning Emily tried an alternative response. Emily was trying to catch up on some work when Dad emerged from his bedroom saying, "I sure would like something from the Big M." She offered to make him something to eat but he said, "Do you want to go get something to eat?" She responded "No, I have a lot of work to do but I would be happy to go for you if you want me to go."

Because of what had happened the day before, Emily wanted Dad to actually *ask* her to go to the Big M for him. She and Dad played cat-and-mouse:

Emily: Do you want me to go for you?
Dad: Do you want to go?
Emily: Only if you want me to. Do you?
Dad: I don't want to bother you.
Emily: It's no bother if you want me to. Do you want me to?
Dad: It's all right, I can walk there. My feet sure hurt today.
Emily: Then if your feet hurt, do you want me to go for you?
Dad: (Reluctantly) All right then, yes.

Did Emily and Dad both win? After all, Dad got his sandwich and she got the response she wanted: Dad asked her to do something for him. Did she feel good about how she handled this situation? No. She was embarrassed to know she had pushed this proud old man to do something she knew he did not want to do.

In looking back, we have tried to analyze our behavior throughout our caregiving. Through this process of retrospection, we concluded, interestingly enough, that certain things our parents said to us when we were teenagers— "you're grounded," "you cannot go out for a week," "go to your room for the rest of the evening," "if you cannot ask for it, it's not worth having," "if you do not hurry up I'm leaving without you," might be considered verbal abuse when an adult child is speaking to an aged parent. While these behaviors were effective in teaching us as children to take responsibility for our actions, they make an already vulnerable adult feel uncomfortable in his or her own home. There is a stage of life, not related to chronological age but to the level of dependency, where the same behaviors take on a new and negative meaning. You have to avoid letting frustration take over so you don't say something you will regret.

The challenge of daily caregiving is exaggerated when what you have done is not acknowledged, even when you consider the frustration the elderly person has to endure. Stay in tune with yourself, your needs versus your wants and your present versus your past. Learn to keep your own cup full and not be dependent on your parent's approval. If keeping your cup full means taking a walk, playing tennis, meditating—do it! Then you are better able to approach challenging situations with a clear head and a gentle expression of your position. You are better able to maintain the sensitivity to understand the elderly person's position; both spoken and unspoken. If successful home care of a parent is to continue, you have to continually reassess and confront the needs, wants and limitation of everyone in the household. Also saying I'm sorry—and meaning it—can help heal hurtful interactions.

My Complements to the Chef

Emily's father, Lank, really enjoyed eating TV dinners because each meal had a nice assortment of meat, potatoes, vegetables and dessert and the portions were small, just what Lank wanted. His taste preference, like my Dad's, were completely different from ours. Because my Dad was showing little interest in eating what Emily prepared, even when she prepared meat and potatoes, we decided to try a couple of Lank's favorite TV dinners on him. Once we prepared dinner we would transfer the meat and potatoes he liked so well to a regular dinner plate and add fresh vegetables and fruit. Often Dad asked, "Who cooked this, Boots?" (Boots is our cousin.) I responded with, "Do you like it?" "Yes!" "Well then, I cooked it." Dad was happy, and complimentary on how well I cooked.

TV dinners helped us get Dad to eat on those days he refused to eat Emily's cooking. The meals are easy to prepare and clean up is a snap. However, TV dinners tend to be high in sodium and since Dad was on a low sodium diet, it was important that we check for sodium levels on the content label and balance the number of TV dinners we prepared in a week with his sausage and biscuit breakfast.

Over time we learned what foods Dad would eat. When Dad becomes bored with both Emily's meals and the TV dinners, we found the local delicatessen a great place to pick up a variety of foods that are not expensive and can be purchased in small quarter pound containers. We'd bring home an assortment of potato, pasta, bean, fruit and Jell-O salads and then add them to a main meat dish.

If your parent wants you to cook a particular food that someone had prepared for him or her years ago, ask how it was prepared and presume nothing. For instance, if a parent told you he or she liked turnips, then refused to eat what you prepared, it could be because of the way it was prepared. Had you known to boil and mash rather than steam and slice the turnips, your parent may have eaten them. When at a complete loss try the supplemental drinks like Ensure. These drinks, found in the pharmacy area of your grocery store, are tasteful and nutritious.

Bank Accounts and Petty Cash

Never separate your parents from their money: by taking control of finances you deprive them of their independence to purchase goods or services. They then have to rely on others to fill basic needs. Take charge of money when parents voluntarily relinquish money handling and bill paying responsibilities, or when they become confused and no longer comprehend money management. If they voluntarily give you responsibility, encourage them to stay active and participate in their money making decisions: don't let them give up—everyone concerned will be better off.

Before Dad was classified homebound, if a relative or friend came to take him for a drive, he would want to share expenses. If he went to a restaurant with someone and he wanted to buy, Dad could do so. If he wanted to travel, buy groceries, clothes or a new pair of glasses, he could. By taking control of his money, we would have deprived him of doing these things for himself. Even when he was unable to go outside, he still liked to treat us to an occasional pizza and he had the money to do it. We cannot imagine any of our parents having to ask us for money for any reason, especially if it belonged to them in the first place.

Of course leaving parents with total control of their money is not without pitfalls. Dad had a history of hiding large sums of money in his residence. We had many concerns about this from his losing interest on savings to potential fire loss. But one of Dad's biggest problems was his inability to remember where he hid money. Some years ago when Dad had to be admitted to the hospital, he told us he had $600 hidden in his wallet somewhere in his apartment but he could not remember where. He had searched every inch of his apartment but could not find it. He assumed it was either stolen or lost for good. One evening, while Emily and I were sitting in the apartment, I was staring at a small hutch in the corner of Dad's living room. I walked over to it and slid my hand along the top of the hutch. The moment I touched it, I knew I'd found his wallet. But a bigger surprise awaited me: when I opened it I found not $600 but twenty-four one hundred dollar bills.

And Dad never changed. One day Dad told me he was getting low on money but when I offered to take him to the bank where he keeps a savings account, he refused. A few days later, he produced a fifty dollar bill for me to pay for items on an errand to the store. Surprisingly, he did not say a word to me about where the money came from. Out of curiosity, I called Dad's bank to see if there had been any withdrawals from his account. Sure enough, three months earlier he had withdrawn

$5,000. Somewhere in the house he had once again hidden his money, only to forget where it was.

There was no reason to mention the pitfalls of hiding money in the house to Dad because he was not going to change. We may not have agreed with what Dad did with his money but it was his to do with as he wished; he earned it. Most certainly, if Dad became disabled or when he died and we decided to dispose of his personal belongings, we determined we would scrutinize, very carefully, everything we discarded. In the meantime, we just had to adjust to the way he wanted to handle his money. But within reason. We would certainly feel more secure if we could have gotten him to keep most of it in a bank.

For all of us money is a negotiating tool. It gives us a sense of autonomy and independence. We can make small purchases such as buying food from the grocery store or we can make major purchases like automobiles. When the elderly give up their money and turn over their financial responsibilities to others, they are disengaging from social, family and financial responsibilities. When this begins to happen, we need to encourage them to stay involved with money matters and concentrate on keeping them as independent as possible for as long as possible. As long as elderly people maintain control of their own money, they maintain control over themselves.

Caregivers Need Rest

It has been our good fortune that our cousins, Edwin and Boots have been enthusiastic "relief" caregivers. Both of them are retired and throughout the year divide their time between Louisiana and Salt Lake City. But we almost missed out on their help because initially we were hesitant to open the door to them. We simply had too little time and too much work to think clearly. When we finally opened that door, we found they were two of the nicest people anyone could ever want for relatives. As my wife likes to say, they are angels. We had little contact with them prior to their moving to Salt Lake City; today we are really good friends. One of their greatest attributes is that they focus a lot of their time on family. Edwin and Boots have shown a great deal of love for our family. Many times, they voluntarily and unconditionally cared for our fathers. When we needed time away from caregiving, Edwin and Boots volunteered to stay with Dad for the day or two we needed to be away. They saw to it that all of his needs were met and they thoroughly enjoyed helping someone who could not do for himself. They did a wonderful job of caregiving and Dad enjoyed the change of pace they introduced to his life.

When we wanted to leave town for more than a few days, we considered hiring a professional aide to come to our home and give round-the-clock care. For us, paying for the vacation and the caregiver was a problem. Another option was separate vacations. One of us could stay home and look after Dad while the other was off vacationing. We were not interested in doing this but it is an option that may work for some couples.

While away, we still maintained daily telephone contact with Dad to include him in what we were doing, making our vacation his in a sense. This gave him something to talk about with his visitors and, more importantly, we knew how Dad was doing.

Hospital stays, while unfortunate for Dad, proved to be beneficial for us. We got caught up on neglected chores, rest and time alone. We never asked anyone to drive Dad to the hospital or return him to his home because we wanted to meet the staff and make sure he was situated and comfortable. We did, on rare occasions, ask friends, relatives and clergy to visit Dad while he was in the hospital. This gave Emily and I the chance to go for a short trip or just spend quiet time at home without feeling like we had abandoned Dad. And, most importantly, we could sleep through the night knowing that while he was in the hospital he was in safe hands.

Dad's time in the hospital provided us respite from constant caregiving, but regardless of whether we stayed at home or left town, we always kept in daily contact with Dad by telephone, just as we did when we went on vacation. We called him to let him know where and what we were doing. This gave him a good feeling of knowing we were doing something we wanted and his daily care was not preventing us from doing it. (It also reminded him that he was important to us, even if we weren't with him.)

Mini-rests are also rejuvenating, like the Mondays when Dad's aide and senior companion came to spend time with him. The five hours the companion spent with him gave us a chance to run errands or do something together.

Also, we decided to have familiar videos available for Dad when we observed how effective "Video Respite" was for the caregivers of Alzheimer's patients. "Video Respite" is being studied at the Gerontology Center at the University of Utah under the direction of Dr. Dale Lund. It involves the value of videos for giving the caregiver time away from the caregiving role. When Dad was feeling good, he really enjoyed railroad videos and videos of his family. When he watched the videos, Emily and I had a couple of hours of "free" time.

Respite options increase for caregivers of parents who are not homebound. For example, senior centers offer congregate lunches on a regular basis. The centers provide a place where the elderly can congregate, not only for lunch but for card playing or just visiting.

Another respite option for non-homebound parents is a visit to large department stores or supermarkets. These stores often have electric carts and they encourage the disabled and the elderly to ride on them. Because these carts are easy for the elderly to drive, they provide caregiver and his or her parent the opportunity to split up in a stimulating and relatively safe environment for both.

We have observed many older people using electric store carts. With no one rushing them, they seem to have an enjoyable time just driving around the stores, shopping and looking at all of the different things on display. Also, going to these stores gives the elderly an opportunity to socialize with whomever they go with or meet. If they get hungry, they can go to the store delicatessen and treat themselves to lunch. A few hours in a store like this can improve the quality of both the parent's and the caregiver's day because the parent gets out of the house and the caregiver gets a break.

The single greatest need for the caregiver is respite—time away from caregiving. It allows you time for yourself and for the things you enjoy, leaving you calm and inspired to meet the daily challenge of long-term caregiving. Organize and plan your time, allowing for the unexpected. Take mini-breaks for yourself and rest when a companion comes to your home; use that time for yourself. Remember, if you schedule time for yourself and the things you enjoy, you will be calm and energized to meet the daily challenge of long-term caregiving.

Because rest for the caregiver is so important, we strongly suggest you do not close the door to people who walk into your life and offer to help. They may provide you with a gift of time as well as enjoyable relationships. When people offer to help, accept graciously and be specific about your needs.

Medicare Insurance

Because Medicare is a very complex system, we touch here on only a small portion of what it entails. Here, we concentrate on helping you understand what you have to do to qualify for Medicare coverage of a short-term nursing home stay. We also discuss what we learned about how the Medicare system works, both internally and externally, while working with medical service providers and insurance companies.

There are two parts to Medicare: Part A and Part B. *Part A* covers hospitalization and related costs for skilled nursing, hospice and home health services following hospitalization. Coverage is measured in benefit periods. A benefit period begins the day you are admitted to a hospital or skilled nursing facility and ends when you have been out of the facility for sixty straight days. A new benefit period begins when you are next admitted to a hospital or care facility.

When I started processing Dad's Medicare forms, I didn't know Medicare is health insurance for people sixty-five and over and is only available to those who paid into the Social Security system through FICA taxes while they worked. I thought every elderly person was eligible. Medicare can be viewed as an eighty percent/twenty percent plan: it pays eighty percent of the covered services and the recipient of services is responsible for the twenty percent balance. This is why it is good to have a secondary insurance that covers the remaining twenty percent. Before your secondary insurance company will pay the remaining twenty percent of the charges, it must have the *Explanation of Your Medicare Part B Benefits* (EOMB) notice. The EOMB allows your insurer to see what charges Medicare approved and how much Medicare has already paid. Medicare sends EOMB notices, which have the words "THIS IS NOT A BILL" printed in the upper right hand corner, to both the patient and the provider of service. If the service provider does not forward the notice to your secondary insurance company, you are responsible for doing so.

The people initially involved in designing Medicare forms forgot one of the basic rules of the written word, "eschew obfuscation" which means "avoid making anything difficult to understand." The forms are often very difficult to understand and often seem contradictory. Based on our experience, I will attempt to clarify these forms in this section.

There is no limit to the number of benefit periods you can have in a year. However, there is a limit to the number of days Medicare will help pay for inpatient hospital or skilled nursing care per year: Part A will help pay for up to 100 days per year. If you exceed the care limit, you are responsible for all charges for each additional day of care until the next year starts.

During the first 60 days of hospital care, Medicare pays all covered costs except a lump sum of $736, the 1996 hospital deductible which is your responsibility. You pay this deductible only once during any given benefit period regardless of the number of times you go to the hospital.

When a person who has been in the hospital is transferred to a nursing home for *skilled nursing care,* Medicare will pay for 100 percent of the first twenty days of nursing home stay. If that same person is released back to their home from the nursing home, he or she must wait for a period of sixty days before Medicare will allow a new benefit period to start. This process can continue until the 100 days of skilled nursing care per year has been used up.

For the first twenty days of the skilled nursing care, Medicare will pay 100 percent of the bill providing the doctor wrote the orders correctly to indicate the patient has spent three consecutive days in the hospital, that skilled nursing care is required *and* that nursing care is directly related to the illness or injury that required the hospitalization.

Starting on the twenty-first day of the stay in the nursing care facility, a co-payment kicks in. For the next eighty days of stay, it is the patient's responsibility to pay the co-payment, $92 per day in 1996 (this co-payment amount increases on a regular basis). If the patient has secondary insurance, the secondary insurance policy should cover most if not all of the $92.

Medicare Part B covers eighty percent of the cost of physician services and physical, occupational and speech therapy services provided by therapists or certain approved institutions and agencies. Part B coverage is subject to a $100 annual deductible and co-insurance is required for full coverage. The co-insurance should cover twenty percent of the Medicare-approved charge.

An EOMB for services provided under Part A will read, "Medicare Benefit Notice — This Is Not A Bill," while the EOMB for services covered under Part B will read, "This Is Not A Bill —Explanation of Your Medicare Part B Benefits." EOMB statements are sent separately for services covered under Part A and under Part B.

We recommend that everyone who qualifies for Medicare have a good backup secondary or supplemental insurance that will pay for the so-called "Medicare Gap," the remaining twenty percent charge Medicare does not cover. Twenty percent of a $40,000 bill is an $8,000 obligation that must be paid. A co-payment in a nursing care facility of $92 per day amounts to quite a large sum of money in a short period of time. A stay of just ten days at that price produces a bill of $920 that Medicare will not cover.

A sample *Explanation of Your Medicare Part B Benefits* notice appears on the following page. The box in the upper right hand corner titled "Summary of this notice dated Jan 15, 1996" shows the total charges of $102.50 and indicates Medicare has approved $27.35. If the figures in this box show that Medicare has not completely reimbursed the provider, look down at the section immediately below in which the various charges are itemized. The column to the far right, headed "See Notes Below," gives letter codes, in this case a, b and c. In the next section, under the heading "NOTES," each letter used in the "See Notes Below" column is paired with an explanation of why Medicare has or has not reimbursed the services provider.

A sample of the form, *Important Information You Should Know About Your Medicare Part B Benefits*, is found following the first Medicare form. This document provides basic guidelines ranging from appealing the amount of a Medicare payment to reducing medical costs.

12345-00011111-00000-1-1-01-02-A-1-A-A-A 0
MEDICARE
MetraHealth Insurance Co.
P. O. Box 123456
S L C, UT 84000

THIS IS NOT A BILL

Explanation of Your Medicare **Part B** Benefits

HARDYN WATSON
1234 ANY STREET
SALT LAKE CITY, UT 84000-0000

Summary of this notice dated January 15, 1996		
Total charges:	$	102.50
Total Medicare approved:	$	27.35
We paid your provider:	$	27.35
Your total responsibility:	$	0.00

Your Medicare Number is: A-111-11-1111

Your provider accepted assignment.

Details about this notice (See the back for more information.)

BILL SUBMITTED BY: ABC LAB
Mailing address: 0000 State Street, SLC, UT 84000

Dates	Services and Service Codes	Charge	Medicare Approved	See Notes Below
	Control number: 00000-0000-00-000			
	ABC LAB			
Dec 11, 1995	1 Urinalysis, nonauto, w/ scope (11111)	$ 14.03	$ 4.47	a,b
Dec 11, 1995	1 Urine culture, colony count (22222)	42.10	10.65	a,b
Dec 11, 1995	1 Antibiotic sensitivity, Mic (33333)	18.87	12.23	a,b
Dec 11, 1995	1 Specimen handling (44444)	+ 27.50	+ 0.00	c
	Total	$ 102.50	$ 27.35	

NOTES:

a Payment for the laboratory test is based on a fee schedule.

b Medicare pays the full approved amount. The deductible does not apply.

c Medicare does not pay for this separately since payment of it is included in our allowance for other services you received on the same day. You cannot be billed separately for this service.

GENERAL INFORMATION ABOUT MEDICARE

Get a mammogram--A picture that can save your life. Your physician or carrier can provide information on this Medicare covered service.

The Medicare Division of The Travelers has become the Medicare Division of MetraHealth Insurance Company. You will notice the MetraHealth name being used in statements or mailings from us. Office locations, phone numbers, and staff members will remain the same.

IMPORTANT: If you have questions about this notice, call the Medicare Division of MetraHealth Insurance Company at 1-800-833-4455 or 1-801-359-0227 or see us at 675 East 500 South, S. L. C., UT. 84102. You will need this notice if you contact us.

To appeal our decision, you must write to us before July 15, 1996. See #2 on the back.

Important Information You Should Know About Your Medicare Part B Benefits

For more information about services covered by Medicare, please see your *Medicare Handbook.*

1. **What should I do if I have questions about this notice?**

   If you have questions about this notice, call, write, or visit us and we will tell you the facts **that** we used to decide what and how much to pay. Turn to the front of this notice; our address and phone number are on the bottom of the page.

2. **Can I appeal how much Medicare paid for these services?**

   If you do not agree with what Medicare approved for these services, you may appeal our decision. To make sure that we are fair to you, we will not allow the same people who originally processed these services to conduct this review.

   However, in order to be eligible for a review, you must write to us within **6 months** of the date of this notice, unless you have a good reason for being late (for example, if you had an extended illness which kept you from being able to file on time).

   Turn to the front of this notice; the deadline date and our address are on the bottom of the page. It may help your case if you include a note from your doctor or supplier (provider) that tells us what was done and why.

   If you want help with your appeal, you can have a friend, lawyer or someone else help you. Some lawyers do not charge unless you win your appeal. There are groups, such as lawyer referral services, that can help you find a lawyer. There are also groups, such as legal aid services, who will give you free legal services if you qualify.

3. **How much does Medicare pay?**

   The details on the front of this notice explain how much Medicare paid for these services. See your copy of *The Medicare Handbook* for more information about the benefits you are entitled to as a beneficiary in the Medicare Part B program. If you need another copy of the handbook, call or visit your local Social Security Office.

   Medicare may make adjustments to your payment. We may reduce the amount we pay for services by a certain percentage (Balanced Budget Law). If your provider accepted assignment, you are not liable to pay the amount of this reduction. We pay interest on some claims not paid within the required time.

   All Medicare payments are made on the condition that you will pay Medicare back if benefits are also paid under insurance that is primary to Medicare. Examples of other insurance are employer group health plans, automobile medical, liability, no fault or workers' compensation. Notify us immediately if you have filed or could file a claim with insurance that is primary to Medicare.

4. **How can I reduce my medical costs?**

   Many providers have agreed to be part of **Medicare's participation program**. That means that they will always accept the amount that Medicare approves as their full payment. Write or call us for the name of a participating provider or for a free list of participating providers.

   A provider who accepts assignment for covered services can charge you only for the part of the annual deductible you have not met and the copayment which is 20 percent of the approved amount.

   If you are treated by one of these doctors, you can save money. See *The Medicare Handbook* for more information about how you can reduce your medical costs.

   Generally a doctor who has not accepted assignment may not charge more than 120 percent of the Medicare approved amount for services provided in 1992, or more than 115 percent for services provided in 1993 or later. This is known as the **limiting charge**. Contact us if assignment was not accepted, and you think your doctor charged more than the limiting charge.

   Some states have laws that could further reduce your medical costs. Please see *The Medicare Handbook* published in 1993 or later for more information.

5. **How can I use this notice?**

   You can use this notice to:

   - Contact us immediately if you think Medicare paid for a service you did not receive;
   - Show your provider how much of your deductible you have met;
   - Claim benefits with another insurance company. If you send this notice to them, make a copy of it for your records.

Keep this notice for your records.
Health Care Financing Administration.

Medicare has many examples of the sorts of explanations that appear in the notes sections of the EOMB form. The examples in this book are taken from our parents' forms and translated from "Medicare-speak" into simpler language. Some of the letter code responses are fairly easy to understand while others require comprehensive explanations. The standard Medicare explanations are in regular type, while our translations are italicized.

> Medicare has established flat rates for reimbursement of facility charges. TRANSLATION: *Medicare has a fee schedule which sets prices for various services. Medicare may make adjustments to your payment. Because of the* Balanced Budget Law, *Medicare may reduce the amount it pays for services by certain percentages. If your provider has agreed to serve Medicare patients, you are not obligated to pay the difference between what Medicare says a service should cost and what the provider usually charges.*

> Another Medicare carrier handles the bills for these services. We have sent the information to them. You will receive a notice from them. TRANSLATION: *There are numerous Medicare insurance carriers such as CIGNA, Travelers and Metropolitan. Medicare uses a variety of letters (assigned when you apply for Medicare benefits) to identify Social Security recipients who receive EOMB notices. For example, the letter A is used to identify all people who worked for the railroad. For example, if the Social Security numbers reads A-111-11-1111, then that person worked for a railroad. So if the patient worked for a railroad and the provider of service sent his bill to the wrong Medicare carrier, that carrier forwards it to the proper Medicare carrier. You eventually will receive an EOMB notice from the railroad Medicare carrier.*

The Medicare number shown on your claim was incorrect or missing. Please ask your provider to use the Medicare claim number shown on this notice on future claims. TRANSLATION: *The provider either omitted your Social Security number or did not copy it correctly onto the bill.*

The amount approved for this more expensive item of durable medical equipment is based on the approved amount for a more standard item. This is the maximum allowable amount for this item. TRANSLATION: *If, for example, you were to purchase the most expensive electric hospital bed available instead of the cheaper, hand-operated model, you would have to pay the difference between the two beds.*

Medicare will make monthly rental payments for the period certified by your doctor. Please notify us immediately if you are no longer using this equipment. TRANSLATION: *If you were to rent a hospital bed rather than purchase one, Medicare would pay rental charges of the approved amount only. You notify Medicare when you are through using the bed.*

This payment is the result of a review of charges previously denied. If you do not agree with what Medicare approved for these services, you may request a review in writing by sending a signed and dated copy of this notice to the address shown below. TRANSLATION: *If you do not agree with what Medicare approved for services, you may appeal its decision. In order to be eligible for a review, you must write to Medicare within a certain period of time from the date of it's notice. Protocol for a review is explained on the opposite side of the EOMB notice page under "Important Information You Should Know About Your Medicare Part B Benefits."*

Medicare will pay for only one hospital visit or consultation per physician per day. You do not have to pay this amount. TRANSLATION: *If you were to visit your physician's office for consultation in the morning and he asked you to return that same afternoon, you could not be charged twice by the physician.*

This is a duplicate of a charge we have processed. TRANSLATION: *A claim has been processed and now Medicare has received another claim for the same charge.*

This service is subject to a reduction of the payment amount. The reduction is ten percent. TRANSLATION: *In this particular situation Medicare has determined, for whatever reason, the provider of service has to reduce the bill by ten percent and it cannot pass that higher charge on to you. It is the responsibility of the service provider to absorb this reduction.*

Your provider did not file this claim within 15 months. You can be billed only twenty percent of the charges that would have been approved by Medicare. TRANSLATION: *This is true even though no Medicare payment can be made.*

It appears you did not know Medicare would not pay for this service so Medicare does not hold you liable. We will pay any amount you have paid your doctor or supplier for the service. To get this payment, submit to this office three things: 1. a copy of this notice; 2. your doctor's or supplier's bill; and 3. a receipt or other proof that you have paid the bill. You should file your written request for payment within 6 months of the date of this notice. Do not apply for this payment if you know Medicare will not pay. TRANSLATION: *A provider must submit it's bill within a certain period of time and if it doesn't you will receive this kind of response from Medicare. If the provider of service does not bill Medicare in a timely manner, that is, within one year, the provider will be penalized financially and you will not be responsible for the difference.*

Medicare cannot pay for this because your provider used an invalid or incorrect procedure code and/or modifier for the service you received. Please ask your provider to resubmit the claim with the valid procedure code and/or modifier TRANSLATION: *You cannot be charged for this service. If you had not read the NOTES on this particular Explanation of Medical Benefits, you would not have been aware that it was your responsibility to contact the provider to inform them they needed to resubmit their bill to Medicare.*

Medicare pays the full approved amount. The deductible does not apply. TRANSLATION: *You have no obligations to pay on this service when this response appears because there is no deductible.*

Payment for the laboratory test is based on a fee schedule. TRANSLATION: *The fee schedule is what sets prices for various services. You cannot be charged the difference between the submitted amount of a bill and the amount Medicare approved.*

Remember, these are but a few of the examples we extracted from our parent's EOMB notices. Read the notes section carefully on every EOMB statement and when in doubt, call Medicare for assistance.

Medicare is currently revising its forms in an attempt to make them more understandable. The sample forms on the following pages are currently being tested in select markets. The new forms do seem to explain more. For example, the notice is now labeled, "Medicare Summary Notice." The phrase, "THIS IS NOT A BILL" is now located at the bottom of the form. *"Keep this notice for you records"* is added to reduce the number of people who think they need to pay the amount shown on the notice. Rather than indicate that a doctor cannot charge more than 115 or 120 percent of Medicare's allowed charge for a certain service, the new form, in the notes section, indicates the limit as a dollar amount. The new "Important Information" section found on the back of the form seems to go into greater detail about what services are and are not covered and warns against Medicare fraud. Don't get the wrong message here: you should still review your Medicare notices very carefully. However, Medicare notices in the future may make this easier to do.

PARTICIPATING/NONPARTICIPATING MEDICARE PHYSICIANS AND SERVICE SUPPLIERS

Medicare uses a number of terms that make their forms and form processing difficult to understand. To make it easier, we will translate some of the "Medicare-speak" terms we encountered into English. A *participating physician* or *supplier* is one who accepts assignment on a Medicare claim. To "accept assignment" means the physician or supplier agrees to accept the amount approved by Medicare as payment for particular services. Medicare will cover eighty percent of the approved charges on a Medicare claim and make payment directly to the provider of service. You are responsible for the deductible and the twenty percent balance of what Medicare approved. *Approved amount* means the amount Medicare determines to be reasonable for a service covered under Part B. The approved amount is taken from a fee schedule that assigns a dollar value to all Medicare-covered services.

A *nonparticipating physician* or *supplier* does not accept assignment on a Medicare claim. When a physician or a supplier does not accept assignment, you must pay the physician

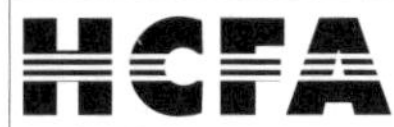

MEDICARE • MEDICAID
Health Care Financing Administration

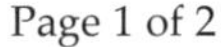

Medicare Summary Notice

June 10, 1996

BENEFICIARY NAME
STREET ADDRESS
CITY, STATE ZIP CODE

CUSTOMER SERVICE INFORMATION
Your Medicare Number: 111-11-1111A

If you have questions, write or call:
Medicare
555 Medicare Blvd.
Suite 200
Medicare Building
Medicare, US XXXXX-XXX

Local: (XXX) XXX-XXXX
Toll-free: 1-800-XXX-XXXX
Tele-Device for the Deaf: 1-800-XXX-XXXX

HELP STOP FRAUD: Beware of telemarketers offering free or discounted Medicare items or services.

This is a summary of claims processed from 5/10/96 through 6/10/96.

PART B MEDICAL INSURANCE-ASSIGNED CLAIMS

Dates of Service	Services Provided	Amount Charged	Medicare Approved	Medicare Paid Provider	You May Be Billed	See Notes Section
Paul Jones, M.D., 123 West Street Jacksonville, FL 33231-0024						**a**
Referred by: Scott Wilson, M.D.						
4/19/96	1 Influenza Immunization (90724)	$5.00	$3.88	$3.88	$0.00	b
4/19/96	1 Admin, flu vac (G0008)	5.00	3.43	3.43	0.00	b
	Claim Total	**$10.00**	**$7.31**	**$7.31**	**$0.00**	
ABC Ambulance, P. O. Box 2149 Jacksonville, FL 33231-0024						
4/25/96	1 Ambulance, base rate (A0020)	$289.00	$249.78	$199.82	$49.96	
4/25/96	1 Ambulance, per mile (A0021)	21.00	16.96	13.57	3.39	
	Claim Total	**$310.00**	**$266.74**	**$213.39**	**$53.35**	

PART B MEDICAL INSURANCE-UNASSIGNED CLAIMS

Dates of Service	Services Provided	Amount Charged	Medicare Approved	Medicare Paid You	You May Be Billed	See Notes Section
William Newman, M.D., 362 North Street Jacksonville, FL 33231-0024						**a**
3/10/96	1 Office/Outpatient Visit (99213)	$47.00	$33.93	$27.15	$39.02	c
Brian Wilson, M.D., 345 18th Street, Jacksonville, FL 33231-0024						**a**
Referred by: Monica Alpert, M.D.						
3/21/96	1 Chest X-ray (71020)	$13.80	$12.04	$9.63	$13.80	

THIS IS NOT A BILL - Keep this notice for your records.

Pt. B Outreach - 9/96

Your Medicare Number: 111-11-1111A

June 10, 1996

Notes Section:

a This information is being sent to your private insurer. They will review it to see if additional benefits can be paid. Send any questions regarding your supplemental benefits to them.

b. This service is paid at 100% of the Medicare approved amount.

c Your doctor did not accept assignment for this service. Under Federal law, your doctor cannot charge more than $39.02. If you have already paid more than this amount, you are entitled to a refund from the provider.

Deductible Information:

You have met the Part B deductible for 1996.

General Information:

If you were offered free items or services but Medicare was billed, please call your local Customer Service at (XXX) XXX-XXXX or toll-free at 1-800-XXX-XXXX.

Appeals Information - Part B

If you disagree with any claim decision on this notice, you can request an appeal by **December 10, 1996**. Follow the instructions below:

- Circle the item(s) you disagree with and explain why you disagree.
- Send this notice, or a copy, to the address in the "Customer Service Information" box on Page 1.
- Sign here ______________________________ Phone number ______________

Pt. B Outreach - 9/96

IMPORTANT INFORMATION
ABOUT YOUR MEDICARE PART B MEDICAL INSURANCE BENEFITS

For more information about services covered by Medicare, please see your *Medicare Handbook*.

MEDICARE PART B MEDICAL INSURANCE: Medicare Part B helps pay for doctors' services, diagnostic tests, ambulance services, durable medical equipment, and other health care services. Medicare Part A Hospital Insurance helps pay for inpatient hospital care, inpatient care in a skilled nursing facility following a hospital stay, home health care and hospice care. You will be sent a separate notice if you receive Part A services or any outpatient facility services.

MEDICARE ASSIGNMENT: Medicare Part B claims may be **assigned** or **unassigned**. Providers who accept **assignment** agree to accept the Medicare approved amount as total payment for covered services. Medicare pays its share of the approved amount directly to the provider. You may be billed for unmet portions of the annual deductible and the coinsurance. You may contact us at the address or telephone number in the Customer Service Information box on the front of this notice for a list of participating providers who always accept assignment. You may save money by choosing a participating provider.

Doctors who submit unassigned claims have not agreed to accept Medicare's approved amount as payment in full. Generally, Medicare pays you 80% of the approved amount after subtracting any part of the annual deductible you have not met. A doctor who does not accept assignment may charge you up to 115% of the Medicare approved amount. This is known as the **Limiting Charge**. Some states have additional payment limits. The NOTES section on the front of this notice will tell you if a doctor has exceeded the Limiting Charge and the correct amount to pay your doctor under the law.

YOUR RESPONSIBILITY: The amount in the "YOU MAY BE BILLED" column is your share of cost for the services shown on this notice. You are responsible for:

- **annual deductible**: the first **$100** of Medicare Part B approved charges each calendar year,
- **coinsurance**: 20% of the Medicare approved amount, after the deductible has been met for the year,
- the amount billed, up to the **limiting charge**, for unassigned claims, and
- charges for services/supplies that are not covered by Medicare. You may not have to pay for certain denied services. If so, a NOTE on the front will tell you.

If you have supplemental insurance, it may help you pay these amounts. If you use this notice to claim supplemental benefits from another insurance company, make a copy for your records.

WHEN OTHER INSURANCE PAYS FIRST: All Medicare payments are made on the condition that you will pay Medicare back if benefits could be paid by insurance that is primary to Medicare. Types of insurance that should pay before Medicare include employer group health plans, no-fault insurance, automobile medical insurance, liability insurance and workers' compensation. Notify us right away if you have filed or could file a claim with insurance that is primary to Medicare.

YOUR RIGHT TO APPEAL: If you disagree with what Medicare approved for these services, you may appeal the decision. You must file your appeal within **6 months of the date of this notice**. Follow the appeal instructions on the front of the last page of this notice. If you want **help with your appeal**, you can have a friend or someone else help you. There are also groups, such as legal aid services, that will provide free advisory services if you qualify. You may contact us for the names and telephone numbers of groups in your area. To contact us, please see our Customer Service Information box on the front of this notice.

HELP STOP MEDICARE FRAUD: Fraud is a false representation by a person or business to get Medicare payments. Some examples of fraud include:

- offers of goods or money in exchange for your Medicare Number;
- telephone or door-to-door offers of free medical services or items, and
- claims for Medicare services or items you did not receive.

If you think a person or business is involved in fraud, you should call Medicare at the Customer Service telephone number on the front of this notice.

INSURANCE COUNSELING AND ASSISTANCE: Insurance Counseling and Assistance programs are located in every State. These programs have volunteer counselors who can give you free assistance with Medicare questions, including enrollment, entitlement, Medigap and premium issues. If you would like to know how to get in touch with your local Insurance Counseling and Assistance Program Counselor, please call us at the number shown in the Customer Service Information box on the front of this notice.

Health Care Financing Administration *Pt. B Outreach - 9/96* for the total charges of the service provided. Medicare will reimburse you eighty percent of what its approved charge is for the particular service. Your out-of-pocket expense will be greater using a nonparticipating service provider. NOTE: While nonparticipating Medicare physicians can charge more than participating Medicare physicians, there is a limit as to the amount they can charge you for services covered by Medicare. By law, they are not permitted to charge more than 115 percent of the Medicare-approved amount for the service.

Before receiving any services or supplies, always ask whether service providers will accept assignment of your Medicare claim even if they do not participate in Medicare. Many nonparticipating providers of services accept assignment on a case-by-case basis. Also, physicians and suppliers are required by law to file your Medicare claim for you regardless of whether or not they accept assignment.

To determine which physicians accept assignment on Medicare claims in your state, contact your Blue Cross/Blue Shield representative and have a Medicare participating physicians/supplier directory (MEDPARD) sent to you. This directory contains the names, addresses, telephone numbers and specialties of Medicare participating physicians and suppliers that have agreed to accept assignment on all Medicare claims for covered items and services. But beware: the directory may not be current. So when you select a physician, call to confirm he or she is still accepting Medicare assignments.

Taking Responsibility for Dad's Insurance

When Dad had surgery in Ohio, I found out he didn't understand anything about how his insurance worked. Instead of soliciting help, in his confusion, he collected the insurance forms and statements as they came in, tossed them in a drawer and did nothing with them.

Whenever I called him to see how he was doing, he would always bring up his medical bills. He had no idea how much he owed or to whom he owed it. He said he had so many statements demanding payment that he did not know what to do. Also, if he received a statement often enough, he paid it and didn't remember to whom or for what. Finally, I told him to send me all of his medical papers, regardless of what they were, and I would sort through them for him. But even after repeated telephone reminders, he would forget to send them. I eventually called Medicare and told them that my father could no longer handle his medical papers. Instead, I requested all his EOMB notices be sent to me.

Before giving me power to receive Dad's medical bills, Medicare needed a signed letter from Dad stating he wanted his son to receive all correspondence from Medicare and to act as his agent. With his approval, I typed up a letter for Dad, had him sign it, then mailed it off to Medicare. After that, all Medicare papers and correspondence came directly to me.

When I started processing Medicare forms for Dad and for my father-in-law, Lank, I had little knowledge of what to do. It was strictly "on-the-job" training. By using my Dad's situation as an example, I will show further frustrations that can be encountered when working with Medicare and secondary insurance companies. Again, I hope my story will spare you some of these same frustrations.

Déjà vu. I found myself in a similar situation to the one I faced processing Lank's insurance forms because I didn't follow specific, detailed steps:

1. When contacting any company concerning medical problems where papers need to be mailed back and forth, get the names of the people with whom you are speaking.

2. Obtain and note in writing for future reference the time and date of your call, as well as the person's

phone number. Each time you call, chances are you will be speaking to a different representative. The reality is, you will probably be starting all over again unless you speak to the person with whom you originally spoke. Be sure to tell him or her you're taking notes. If the person with whom you speak knows you are writing down all pertinent information, that person will more likely follow through with your problem the first time. If not, you will be able to remind him or her of the exact time and date you spoke.

3. Always make sure the necessary forms are filled out completely and correctly to begin with and always make copies of what you send.

By ignoring these steps, I got caught again in a maze. Several time-wasting scenarios engulfed large chunks of my days. If the provider of services left the responsibility to Dad for billing his secondary insurance company, the insurance forms had to be filled out right the first time or we had problems. For instance, while I attached the original EOMB notice to the original secondary insurance form, then mailed them to the secondary insurance company, Dad was receiving statements from different providers of service demanding payment. I contacted the insurance company and was informed they had never received a payment request from the service provider. I then called the provider and requested another insurance form and contacted Medicare for another copy of the EOMB notice. I attached the EOMB notice to the secondary insurance form and mailed it to the secondary insurance company. Delinquent statements continued to arrive; the service providers were still not being paid. I called the insurance company and they still had not received any statements so, once again, they asked me to resubmit the papers. Since I hadn't made copies of the two forms, I had to spend additional time, effort and expense in having new forms sent to me.

This time, however, I sent everything to Dad's secondary insurance via registered mail (signature requested). But whoever accepted the forms penned initials on the signature card and I had no way of identifying that person. The irony here is that later the insurance company told me they had never received the signature-required envelope and requested I repeat the process. Fortunately this time I had made copies.

I learned it was important to read every EOMB notice in its entirety. If there was any part of the notice I didn't understand, I called Medicare and asked questions. If I received a statement from a service provider stating we were delinquent in paying a bill and I had not received an EOMB notice, I called that provider and, on their bill, wrote down the date and time and the name of the person with whom I spoke. My first question to that person was, "Has Medicare been billed?" If the person said yes, I asked "Has Medicare paid their portion?" If the answer was no to either of these questions, then I would wait until Medicare paid. Once Medicare paid, then I asked if a secondary or supplemental insurance had paid its part and, if the answer was no, I asked if they have been billed. If the answer was no, I requested that they bill the insurance company and then I waited until the insurance company had paid.

Finally, I waited for a final statement from the provider that would show me the remaining balance after both Medicare and our secondary insurance had paid. Dad's balance was always relatively low because he had secondary insurance coverage.

We found by the time service providers billed Medicare and the secondary insurance carrier, at least four to six months will have elapsed. If a service provider is waiting for payment from any insurance company, whether it be Medicare or secondary or supplemental insurance, we suggest delaying payment until each insurance company has paid its portion; however, we suggest you take the responsibility to follow up with the insurance companies to make sure the bills are paid. After all, your parents received the services and the bill is their responsibility, not the insurance company's.

Eventually, it becomes easier to know if Medicare has or has not paid the provider because both you and the provider will receive a copy of the EOMB notice. Normally the provider will contact Medicare to see what the delay is when they have not received payment. However, there have been times when providers have asked me to follow up with Medicare and I have.

By communicating with service providers you accomplish two things. First, you know whether the insurance companies have paid or not. Second, you develop a working relationship with the providers and they appreciate the fact that you are not trying to avoid them. We found that when you call service providers, they are willing to work with you.

Many elderly patients who receive itemized statements from their medical provider believe they need to pay the statement as soon as they receive it even though the phrase, "THIS IS NOT A BILL" is printed on it. A combination of poor concentration and bad eye sight can contribute to lack of comprehension. Many service providers unintentionally confuse their patients by sending statements accompanied with a self-addressed return envelope. The sample document, XYZ Physicians Office, on the following page demonstrates how confusing this paperwork can be. The statement shows a balance of $268.17 and a self-addressed envelope was included with the statement. Also notice that at the bottom of the page, the statement shows:

Total Acct Balance of	$268.17
Amount Pending Ins. of	$268.17
Due By Patient Now:	$ .00

Page No. 1

XYZ Physician's Office
000 West Avenue Suite Y
Salt Lake City UT 84000
Billing Only: (801) 000-0000

THIS IS A STATEMENT OF YOUR ACCOUNT ON THE BELOW DATE. ANY CHARGES OR PAYMENTS MADE AFTER THIS DATE WILL APPEAR ON NEXT MONTH'S STATEMENT.

ACCOUNT NO.	STATEMENT DATE
1111	11/30/95

Hardyn Watson
1234 Any Street

Salt Lake City UT 84000

A FINANCE CHARGE of 1.5 % PER MONTH equal to an ANNUAL PERCENTAGE RATE of 18 % PER ANNUM will be added to the unpaid balance of _______ days or more past due as of the billing date appearing on this statement. Payments and other credits are deducted from the Previous Balance before computing the FINANCE CHARGE.

*** ITEMS MARKED WITH AN ASTERISK (*) HAVE BEEN BILLED TO YOUR INSURANCE.

TO INSURE PROMPT CREDIT TO YOUR ACCOUNT, PLEASE DERTACH AND RETURN THIS TOP PORTION OF YOUR STATEMENT WITH YOUR PAYMENT.

DATE	PROCEDURE	POS	CPT	PATIENT NAME	DIAG. CODE	DOCTOR		AMOUNT
	Balance Forward							244.17
11/13/95	Established Pt., Lev	11	00000	HARDYN	111.1	Smith	*	68.00
11/13/95	Venipuncture	11	00000	HARDYN	111.1	Smith	*	8.00
11/13/95	Additional Hemagre	11	00000	HARDYN	111.1	Smith	*	8.33
11/13/95	CBC Auto and Hemogra	11	00000	HARDYN	111.1	Smith	*	12.65
11/13/95	Clinical Chemistries	11	00000	HARDYN	111.1	Smith	*	21.25
11/13/95	Vincristine Sulfate	11	00000	HARDYN	111.1	Smith	*	53.00
11/14/95	Payment - ABC Med			HARDYN		Brown		-181.27
11/14/95	XYZ HEALTH			HARDYN		Brown		-9.70
11/14/95	XYZ HEALTH			HARDYN		Brown		-20.41
11/14/95	XYZ HEALTH			HARDYN		Brown		-6.40
11/14/95	XYZ HEALTH			HARDYN		Brown		-2.98
11/14/95	XYZ HEALTH			HARDYN		Brown		-2.71
11/14/95	XYZ HEALTH			HARDYN		Brown		-8.00
11/14/95	XYZ HEALTH			HARDYN		Brown		-12.70

XYZ Physician's Office

Total Acct. Balance:	268.17
Amount Pending Ins.:	268.17
Due By Patient Now:	.00

Aging:	CURRENT	31 - 60	61 - 90	91 - 120	121 - up
	.00	.00	.00	.00	.00

** Statement Due upon Receipt * Thank You **

Even though this section shows the patient does not owe anything, "Statement Due Upon Receipt. Thank You. " is still printed on the bottom of the page. It's easy to see how some elderly person would pay this bill if he or she were to receive this statement. Most bills are computer generated with these standard phrases and envelopes included. The lesson here is read the bill thoroughly.

We found that by the time service providers bill Medicare and the secondary insurance, at least four to six months will have elapsed.

Now look at the notice from XYZ Medical Center. The notice shows "Amount Due $13.45" again with the statement, "PAYMENT DUE UPON RECEIPT." The idea this is a bill is enforced by the following statement which appears at the bottom of the form:

THIS STATEMENT IS FOR INFORMATIONAL PURPOSES.
PLEASE REMIT ANY OUTSTANDING CO-PAYMENTS, DEDUCTIBLES
OR NON-COVERED CHARGES AT THIS TIME.

Note that the phrase, "For Information Purposes" is immediately followed by a request for remittance. Would you pay this statement? Maybe. We think so because the "informational statement" gets lost among the remittance request and the balance due.

The biggest headache in the matter of insurance is how time-consuming the phone calls become. When I called the hospital to find out if this notice was a bill that needed to be paid, here's what happened. The hospital operator rang Accounts Payable. The woman in Accounts Payable said I needed to speak with Patient Accounting and she gave me that number. At eleven in the morning I began calling the number the operator had given me. No one answered even though I called repeatedly until noon. I figured that whoever was taking calls would be out to lunch until one, so I waited until then before continuing. At 2:40 p.m., I again called but there was

XYZ MEDICAL CENTER
5678 Any Street
Salt Lake City, Utah 84000

Return this stub with payment

We honor VISA, MASTER CARD, and AMERICAN EXPRESS

PAYMENT IS DUE UPON RECEIPT

Admissions	Patient Name
0123456789	WATSON, H G

Unpaid balance from prev. billing	Agreement AMOUNT	Amount Due
		13.45

PLEASE PAY THIS AMOUNT

CHARGE ☐ VISA ☐ MC ☐ AMEX

CARD NUMBER (ALL DIGITS PLEASE)

☐☐☐☐☐☐☐☐☐☐☐☐☐☐☐☐☐☐☐

☐☐☐☐ INTERBANK NUMBER (Master Card Only)

Expiration Date: ______________________

____
SIGNATURE — CHARGE CUSTOMERS ONLY

Hardyn Watson
1234 Any Street
Salt Lake City UT 84000

Address changed? Please make changes above.

Admission No.	Patient Name	Service or Discharge Date
0000000	WATSON, HARDYN G	07/14/95

Date	Description	Amount
	BEGINNING BALANCE	67.25
08/03/95	MEDICARE O/P C/A	35.64-
08/03/95	MEDICARE B PAYMENT	18.16-
	****THIS STATEMENT IS FOR INFORMATIONAL PURPOSES** PLEASE REMIT ANY OUTSTANDING CO-PAYMENTS, DEDUCTIBLES OR NON-COVERED CHARGES AT THIS TIME.**	

Billing Date	Estimated Insurance	Account Balance	Finance Charge	New Balance
12/14/95	13.45	13.45		13.45

Payments received after this date will appear on next statement

A FINANCE CHARGE IS COMPUTED BY A "PERIODIC RATE" OF WHICH IS AN ANNUAL PERCENTAGE RATE OF APPLIED TO THE ADJUSTED ACCOUNT BALANCE, WHICH IS THE PREVIOUS BALANCE LESS CURRENT PAYMENTS AND/OR CREDITS. TO AVOID ADDITIONAL FINANCE CHARGES, PAY THE "NEW BALANCE."

still no answer. I called the hospital operator back and told him my story. He said it was likely that there was only one person working in that department and whoever it was would be taking calls in the order in which they were received.

Since I was at my desk working, I decided to make one last call and just let the telephone ring to see how long it would be before someone finally answered. The phone rang continuously for twenty minutes and still no one answered. Once again, I called the operator and this time I asked to speak with the hospital administrator. A woman who worked in the administrator's office told me the administrator was not available and offered to help me instead. I explained I had been calling Patient Accounting for the past three hours and no one had picked up the phone. She asked what number Accounts Payable had given me and I told her. She put me on hold and in less than a minute she was back on the telephone. She said the Accounts Payable people were using an old directory and had given me the wrong number. She apologized and said she would contact that department and see to it that they gave out the correct numbers in the future. She then very nicely answered my questions. She said this statement was not a bill that needed to be paid; it was a statement letting us know that Dad still had a responsibility to the hospital for $13.45 until his secondary insurance paid it. Even her verbal explanation made it sound like he needed to pay the bill, that it was his responsibility.

Would your elderly parents have called all day to see if they needed to pay this statement or would they have just paid it? The lesson to be learned here is that it may be important for you to intervene on your parent's behalf in his or her insurance matters. Remember, persistence and careful attention to detail can save a lot of headaches.

HOME FOR CHRISTMAS

As Autumn turned to Winter 1996, Dad increasingly spoke of returning to Kentucky so he could be on the hill with his mommy and poppy for Christmas. My once strong 92-year-old father was hallucinating frequently. It was heart-wrenching to see and hear Dad, now small, frail and dying, occasionally crying out for his mommy and poppy. Dad was loosing his ability to think and speak intelligently and was confused about his surroundings and who was with him. He often spoke as though someone was conversing with him and when questioned, would give the name of someone who had died years before. When asked where he thought he was, Dad would say, "On the hill," meaning back home in Kentucky. Just two months earlier, Dad had become focused on going back to Kentucky but we believed there was no way he could make the trip East. Little did we know he would be home for Christmas: Dad was dying.

In mid-November Dad's health began a drastic plunge. He developed another urinary infection with four strains of bacteria, none of which were responding to any antibiotic. Dad's health was deteriorating so rapidly, Emily and I decided to have an early family Thanksgiving dinner. We invited a combination of family and friends we hoped Dad would enjoy. Just a few days before the planned dinner, we had to cancel because neither my Dad nor my Mom, who still lived in Salt Lake, were feeling well. Emily found Mom lying on the bedroom floor of her home, conscious but unable to get up. X-rays revealed four compressed fractures of the vertebrae which meant Mom had to stay in the hospital for the next two weeks.

Meanwhile, Dad's situation continued to worsen. He had neither the interest nor the strength to do the things he enjoyed and no longer wanted to eat or drink or go anywhere. He just wanted to sleep. Finally, because of the difficulty in getting Dad out of bed and because having him sit in a chair was so difficult and seemed to cause him so much pain, we decided to let him remain in bed and just turn him every two hours. Dad stopped taking in any liquid or food over the next two days. Then four days before Christmas, we were unable to wake him in the morning. We told Dad's physician that Dad appeared to be dying and requested a hospice team be sent to our home. It was Saturday; the doctor agreed to make arrangements first thing Monday morning.

Meanwhile, Emily fought with her emotions about whether to call her priest to pray for Dad; neither my father nor I are Catholic. While she was concerned about what I might feel, Emily gave in to her need and called her priest. She told Father Cassian my father was probably in the last stage of life and she would appreciate it if he came to our home and prayed. Father Cassian arrived within the hour, and he and Emily immediately went into Dad's room. Emily went to the side of Dad's bed, took his hand and began rubbing his arm as Father Cassian said, "Hardyn, this is Father Cassian. I met you a couple of times when I was over for dinner here at Emily and George's and I want to say a prayer for you as you continue on with this part of life's journey." He blessed Dad and read a prayer for the sick. "God forgives you all your sins and He is love. He will be with you on this part of the journey and Emily and George are with you." Father Cassian anointed Dad with holy oil and made the sign of the cross on Dad's forehead and asked Emily to join him in saying the Lord's Prayer. Then Father Cassian, with a great deal of emotion and tears in his eyes said, "Goodbye Hardyn. The peace of the Lord be with you." When Emily told me what had taken place, I was pleased Father Cassian responded to her call because I knew how important it had been for Emily and for Dad to have him there.

Emily and I had been sitting vigil throughout the day and into most of the evening. We had rented our basement apartment a year after Lank died, and the two of us were invited downstairs by our tenant for some food and drink. Since we needed a break, we placed Dad's tape player next to his bed and played a soothing Kenny G. musical, a favorite of his. We went downstairs and, after a short stay, we went back up to be with Dad. When we walked into his room, we noticed he was breathing in long intervals. I noticed there was a slight amount of mucus in his mouth; to remove it I pressed a small wet sponge against the back of his throat and he appeared to like that. I placed the wet sponge on Dad's throat a second time, he exhaled once and I realized he was going. I told Emily to take his hand and I took the other one and as we said good-bye, he exhaled one last time. There was no question in our minds, Dad waited for us to be with him before he died, just as Lank had.

Dad died December 21, 1996 of congestive heart and acute renal failure. I noted Dad's time of death and notified a local funeral home. Out of respect for Dad, Emily and I prepared his body one last time before the mortuary staff arrived. As we had done earlier with Lank, we washed and creamed Dad's body. Since he always wanted to be buried in pajamas, we used the bottoms of a pair he saved for this occasion and a new pajama top Byron sent him for Christmas. We placed Dad's dentures in his mouth, put his glasses on his face, placed a ring on a finger of each hand and put his watch on his left wrist.

Some people feel the Christmas season is a terrible time for a death. While the separation and void Dad was leaving in our hearts was difficult to accept, we knew we would be surrounded by friends and family during this special time. We believe when we celebrate Christmas in the future, Dad's death will bring back fond memories of the way he was. Christmas, the mass for Christ, gives such strong support, even a stronger support when we realize God has joined us and is with us in our humanity. Knowing life continues helps us balance our emotions. The holidays provide an overwhelming support which isn't always there at other times of the year. While we are sad because we have seen a man go so far away from where he was, it is still a time for celebrating a life. Emily and I will celebrate the 21st of December from this day on, not because of Dad's death, but for his life.

On a Hill Far Away

The final responsibility of caregivers is seeing to it their parents are buried or cremated according to their wishes. With this responsibility in mind, I contacted the funeral home in Vanceburg, Kentucky, where Dad had his pre-paid funeral agreement, notified the staff there of his death and provided the name and phone number of the Salt Lake City funeral home that was tending to Dad at this end. The Vanceburg staff arranged for Dad to be flown to Cincinnati where they would pick him up and return him to their place for burial preparation. Our expense was $1,140, which arose only because Dad's agreement did not include out-of-state body preparation. The Vanceburg funeral home placed free obituaries in local newspapers and had announcements made on the radio: an additional service we hadn't expected but found effective in notifying people in small rural towns of Dad's funeral.

Since Dad was to be buried in Kentucky and because most of the people he knew here were now dead, we did not place an obituary in the Salt Lake papers; however, we did notify, by phone, a few close relatives and friends. Dad's body flew out of Salt Lake City on December the 23rd. Because of the Christmas holiday and the traveling distance for many of our friends and relatives, Byron and I decided to hold the viewing, memorial service and graveside service all together six days later. Byron and his son John met Emily and me at the Cincinnati airport the day before the funeral. We rented an automobile and drove to Vanceburg.

Before we checked into our motel, we went to the funeral home to make sure everything was in order. John, at thirty-two years old, had never seen a dead person before, so we discussed what he could expect when he saw his grandfather and how Dad's body was only a shell that held his spirit; the true Hardyn was gone to a far better place than he had ever been before. When we arrived for the funeral the next morning, Emily, John and I went to the back of the building where the viewing and services were to be held. Byron elected to stay in the front section of the home and greet people as they arrived. For personal reasons, Byron did not wish to see his Dad in a coffin; he wanted to remember Dad as he had last seen him, content, happy and alert. We all respected Byron's decision. Everyone has his or her own way and timeframe for dealing with death. Although ways may be different, these ways need to be respected

Dad had asked for a simple funeral and we strove to honor his wish. Our cousin Bob Watson eloquently gave a prayer and a few words on Dad's behalf. I spoke a few words of thanks and read a letter Dad's aide wrote when he learned of Dad's death. Dad's humor touched many people in many ways, as shown in the aide's letter:

Dear George and Emily,

I just wanted to write you and thank you for the opportunity I had to take care of your father. He was one of my favorite clients. He always had a smile and I always looked forward to the visits to your home. The visits will be missed.

Your Dad always was trying to "get my goose." He made my job fun. His one-liners made me laugh. "Clean as a hound's tooth," was a favorite. His collections of different items were interesting to see. He told me of friends of his that had served in the Civil War. His recall of events and people in his life amazed me. I don't think I'll ever be able to put another client's glasses on without wanting to call them, "gold rimmed testicles." He was such a good friend.

Darrin

At graveside, Bob Watson again gave a prayer. Then Byron walked to Dad's casket and said he would like to say a few words. He thanked everyone for attending the graveside service and spoke of our fulfilling our commitment to see that Dad was buried where he had always wanted to be, on the hill next to his mommy and poppy. Because Dad always liked and recited poetry, Byron chose to close the services by reading a poem he believed Dad had never heard but would have liked.

Do not stand at my grave and weep.
I am not there. I do not sleep.
I am a thousand winds that blow.
I am the glints on snow.
I am the sunlight on ripened grain.
I am the gentle autumn rain.

When you awaken in the morning's hush,
I am the swift uplifting of quiet birds in circling flight.
I am the soft star that shines at night.
Do not stand at my grave and cry.
I am not there. I did not die.

—Anonymous

Dad would have been proud.

George's Mother

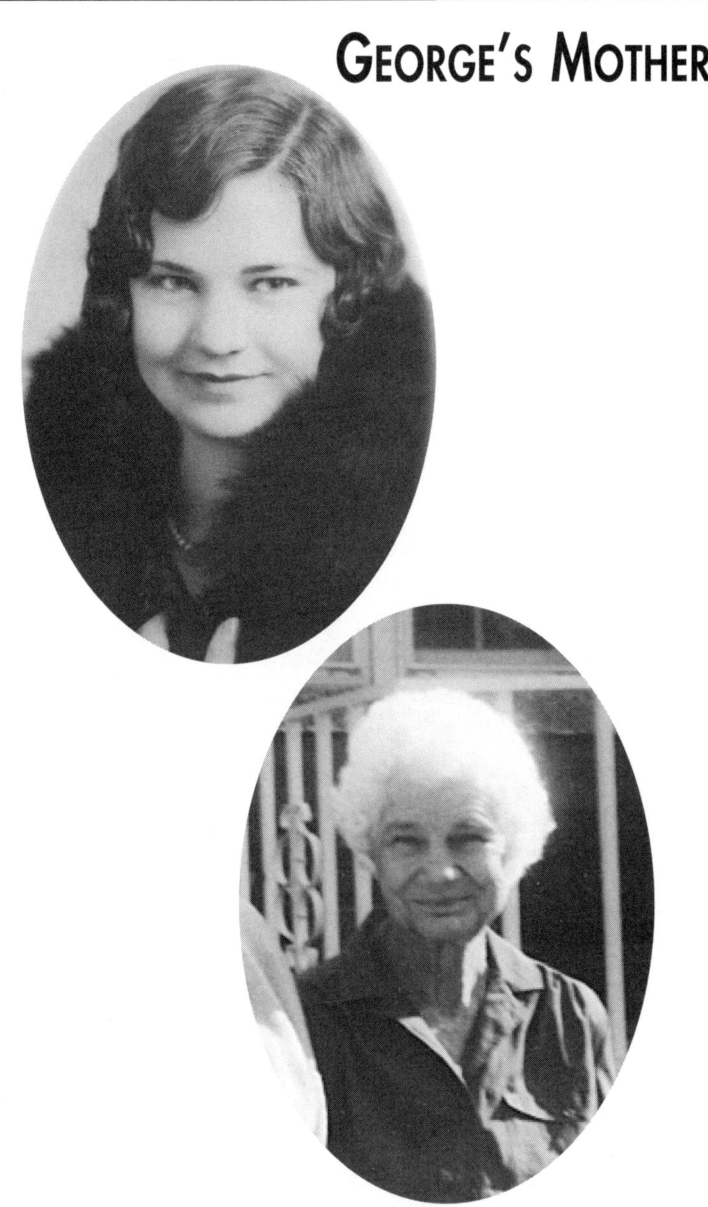

Hazel Elizabeth Cravens Watson

September 4, 1909 — January 16, 1997

My mother Hazel was a beautiful woman when she was a young lady. When she aged she became even more beautiful, both in looks and as a person. Her life with my father was not an easy one: although he was very much in love with her, Hardyn's jealousy caused them both grief. He was prepared to fight any man who looked at Mom twice. In their early and middle years, my parents traveled extensively throughout the United States but as Dad neared retirement they began to drift apart. They eventually started taking separate vacations. In 1970, my mother and father, after forty-three years of marriage, went their separate ways. Mom stayed in our home and Dad moved to Ohio.

Sometime in the early '60s, Mom had quit her sales position with Sears & Roebuck after working there for fifteen years. Since she had paid into the FICA system, she qualified for early Social Security benefits. Her only source of income after the divorce was her Social Security. Mom was fortunate: she could stay in her own home because it was paid for. Had she needed to find another place, she would have had few options. She probably would have moved in with one of her sons.

Mom had been a light smoker when she was married. When she divorced, she graduated to one pack or more per day. Mom's smoking irritated those around her but did not appear to have an adverse effect on her: for the last twenty years of her life Mom's health had been fair to good. While she had been able to do her daily living activities (ADLs), bathing, dressing and cooking, she had limitations in what she could do. Over time I took on the responsibility of doing what she no longer could.

Mom used to drive but for health reasons had to quit. Although she enjoyed mowing, raking and watering her grass, she lost the ability to do those chores. Emily and I took Mom to the grocery store, beautician, senior citizen's dances and did house maintenance repairs, all on Friday, a day we had pretty much dedicated to her. It was a one hour round-trip drive from her house to where she danced. By the time we picked her up and saw her home, it was 11:30 at night.

This Friday routine went on for twenty years. Then, while taking gerontology classes at the university, we found out about the Aging Service's Senior Companion program. We placed Mom's name on a waiting list. Two years later, she got herself a companion. This person visited her for four hours every Friday. Her companion took her to the grocery store and beauty salon, relieving us of these trips, but he did not take Mom to the weekly dance or do chores around her house. We still did these tasks.

If Emily and I wanted—or needed—time off on Friday, we gave Mom advance notice, giving her time to make other arrangements. On rare occasions when we were unable to take Mom someplace she wanted to go, relatives came to her aid and volunteered to take her. Cousins stopped by weekly, taking her fruit or 'just to chat. The LDS Relief Society ladies as well as neighbors also paid regular visits.

Mom was a very independent senior. Even though she lived alone, she did not lack company. Unless some emergency arose, our Friday schedule and daily telephone contact were sufficient to meet her personal needs.

Protecting Mom From Herself

As soon as you start a single maintenance responsibility on a continual basis, realize that you are starting the caregiving role. It is at this time, not at a later undefined date, you want to place your parent's name on the Community Services Council waiting list for yard care or house maintenance services because it could literally take years before volunteer help is available. Furthermore, as our older population increases, that waiting period is sure to increase.

We placed Mom on the waiting list for Assist Services and for Chore Services, the latter a program of the local Community Service Council. Both are private, not-for-profit organizations funded by various municipalities throughout the state of Utah. Neither charge for their services but do ask for donations. During the two years we waited for her to become eligible for these services, Emily and I were involved in daily home-care for both our fathers so by the time Mom started receiving yard and snow service from Chore, we were grateful to be relieved of those duties.

Some elderly people are reluctant to relinquish the care of their home to others but if they are continuously trying to do something that is dangerous to their well-being, you need to step in and make decisions that will ensure their safety. Before Mom was accepted for yard and snow removal services, I became increasingly concerned about her insistence she cut her own grass. Mom was in her mid-70s. She was starting to hunch over and lean to one side. She showed signs of osteoporosis. She would lose her balance in her house and grab for anything—table, chair, wall—to catch herself. I worried because she was still using a large, heavy gas driven lawn mower. If she were to slip and fall, the mower was capable of doing her great bodily harm. I shared my concerns with Mom and although she did not concur, she agreed to allow us to take care of her yard for a one month trial. As it turned out, she enjoyed the extra visit we made to cut the lawn.

When Chore took over her yard duties, initially she was pleased but she soon started to complain the volunteers were mowing her grass at eight in the morning which was too early because she didn't get up until ten. Then when two weeks would elapse without the grass being cut, due to rain or lack of volunteers, she again found reason to complain. Mom did not think of these services as a volunteer effort. She saw them as an entitlement and became extremely critical of how and when they helped her. (At times she was equally critical with us and what we did for her).

The year we took over her yard work, we also found it necessary to remove her snow shovel. Mom was a very impatient person: instead of waiting for us, she would have her walks shoveled before we arrived to do them. She then proceeded to complain about how sore she was. One evening a large snow storm hit the Salt Lake City valley. It snowed all night. The next morning Mom went outside to shovel snow. The snow was deep, the wind biting cold and the temperature in the low teens. Even though her hands were extremely cold, she continued to shovel, this time without wearing gloves. When through, to get her hands warm, she ran hot water over them and instantly they began to sting and burn. She telephoned, telling me what she had done and within ten minutes of her call, her hands had already begun to blister.

We went to InstaCare, where she was treated for frostbite and then released. She no longer realized that when she placed her cold, perhaps frozen, hands under hot water, she risked severe burns. She could have lost fingers. She was, as of that episode, out of the snow removal business. Mom learned to wait.

While Emily and I became frustrated with Mom's lack of appreciation for the volunteer help she was receiving, we still got caught up in her anger of how a job was or was not completed. After a reactive period we would remind her and ourselves, that these people were volunteers who have jobs, family and a home to care for and they were just trying to make her life a little easier.

Don't fret and fume over a free service. Services such as Chore and Assist do not exist to eliminate someone's chores. They exist because there are people who care and want to help provide relief where relief is needed. We were grateful for the assistance Mom received from Assist and Chore. Over a six year period, Chore shoveled snow, cut grass and performed other yard care at Mom's house. Assist took care of Mom's plumbing, cement work, roof repair, painting (inside and out); they replaced a broken water heater and toilet. If Mom used a wheelchair and had needed a handicap railing at her home, Assist would have built one.

How could anyone ask for more, especially when resources are limited and services are free? The volunteers are courteous and conscientious people. We must all do our part when we can to make these programs even more successful. In Salt Lake City, Assist is listed in the business section of the phone book or you can find it through Aging Services/Outreach-Information and Referral Services. Chore Service is listed under the Community Services Council in the business section of the Salt Lake City phone book. Different states will have different names for such programs. Look under Aging Services in the government section.

Anyone can become a volunteer, especially when we find ourselves far from a needy family member. Take a closer look at the needs of someone living near you. You can attempt to meet the challenge of service by looking next door, down the block, or around your neighborhood. Helping with one chore can greatly enhance the quality of someone's day. Remove trash cans from a side yard to the street on collection day, then return them. Place a newspaper, thrown on a porch, at a more reachable level for someone having trouble bending. Mow a lawn. Pick weeds. Shovel snow. Paint something. Help adjust a TV. Grocery shop. Change a light bulb. The list is endless and the need is great.

MEANS-TESTED PROGRAMS

The Area Agency on Aging is designated by the state to address the needs and concerns of all older Americans. Know that specific names of local Area Agencies on Aging may vary. Also, this agency may not be available in every community. Many agencies can be found in the government listings of the telephone directory or the yellow pages under "aging," "senior citizens service organizations" or "social services." These agencies are responsible for a geographic area—either a city, a single county or a multi-county district. They coordinate services including transportation, community-based and in-home services and services for residents in long-term care facilities. Locating these programs and sorting through the qualifications may be time consuming, but they will save your parent money and perhaps be the key to allowing them to stay in their own home.

Once you identify available programs, find out whether or not they are "means-tested." Eligibility for means-tested programs is determined by the amount of cash and assets you own: the less you have, the greater the chance of qualifying for these programs. Assets, in most cases, include anything you can sell or use to take care of yourself. They include but are not limited to real estate, antiques, vehicles and money in the bank.

Qualified Medicare Beneficiary (QMB) is a means-tested insurance program. Because Mom did not have secondary insurance, we contacted the Office of Family Support and made an appointment to meet with an adviser to determine if Mom was eligible for QMB benefits, an insurance that shares the patient's medical cost with Medicare. It pays the twenty percent of medical services that Medicare does not pay. It is for people like my Mom — over sixty with limited income and assets. While the program is means-tested, each state probably has different guidelines for qualification.

Mom's only income was her Social Security check, which was under the $665 qualifying monthly limit: her savings was also under a single person's allowable amount of $4000 (for a couple the qualifying amount was $6,000 as of 1996). Owning a home will not necessarily disqualify someone from getting QMB coverage. So, if your parents own their own home, but don't have a secondary insurance policy and have meager assets, don't give up. Find out what the qualifications are for your state. A person must qualify once a year and a QMB medical card is issued each month because Medicaid, which pays the premium, is a month-by-month program. The medical card must be presented to the service provider at the time services are requested.

In Utah, contact numbers for the Family Support Office which administers the QMB program, are located in the State Government section of the telephone book under Human Services, Department of Family Support Office. To locate the QMB office in your area, dial 1-800-677-1116, or call Aging Services or the health department.

Another secondary insurance source that should be considered is the "Specified Low-Income Medicare Beneficiary" (SLMB) program. It is for persons entitled to Medicare Part A whose incomes are slightly higher than the national poverty level. The program only pays Medicare Part B premiums. The monthly income limits for the SLMB program in 1996 for all states except Alaska and Hawaii were $794 for an individual and $1,057 for a couple. For more information contact your state or local Medicaid, public welfare or social services office.

In addition to insurance, there are means-tested tax programs. If people whose sole income is from Social Security were forced to pay all property taxes on their homes, it would probably force many of them to sell their homes and find a new place to live. There is relief available through state means-tested tax programs. To receive tax relief a person must meet the requirements of limited assets, advanced age or have a sight disability. Contact the county treasurer for an application for exemption and/or credit on property tax.

Another program available for the elderly is the Office of Family Support's "HEAT" program (Home Energy Assistance Target) which is offered through the Department of Human Services. HEAT helps defray the cost of winter heat bills for those who qualify. Each state has a similar program. Call the Department of Human Services or your local fuel companies for instructions on how to apply for this assistance.

MEDICAID

We discuss Medicaid only briefly because it is a complex program and it seems as if some of the rules change monthly. Medicaid is a federally funded state matching program that provides basic health care for the elderly poor. It is a means-tested benefit rather than an entitlement. Medicaid is only available for people sixty-five or older, blind, or formally classified as disabled who cannot afford their own health care costs. Medicaid favors care in institutions. It does not pay for services outside of the nursing home and has nothing to do with home health care. Medicaid does pay for long-term care but only for those who are poor or who have become impoverished because of high nursing home costs.

Medicaid has financial qualifications: on the day of admission to a long-term care facility, a single individual must have countable assets of less than $2000. Countable assets include everything you can sell or use to take care of yourself including real estate, stocks, bonds and money in the bank. Other assets are not "countable" or exempt including the person's home, household and personal goods and one vehicle (if its value doesn't exceed a certain limit).

To receive assistance from Medicaid for nursing home services, an individual must have a medical need to be in the nursing home and must qualify financially as well. An individual must meet two out of the following three nursing home criteria:

Activities of Daily Living Deficit—Assistance is required with any one of the following: bathing, feeding, ambulation (walking), taking medications, dressing, grooming or transfers (wheelchair to bed).

Cognitive Deficit —The person is completely disoriented, that is to say, he or she does not know who anyone is, what time of day or night it is or where he or she is. The person has short- term and long-term memory loss.

Bowel and Bladder Deficit —The person is incontinent, unable to control bowel and/or bladder function.

If a person owns countable assets that exceed $2000, a "spend down" must take place in order to qualify for Medicaid. It is important for everyone to understand how spend down works. For example, the total amount of assets a married couple can have is $145,320. Divided equally, each spouse's share is $72,660. The spouse who will live in the nursing home must "spent down" his or her half to $2000 before being eligible for Medicaid.

It is illegal and fraudulent to hide funds or to apply for Medicaid based on false or misleading information. So don't do it. When applying for Medicaid, honesty is the best policy. Do not assume Medicaid does not care about any particular asset; you will likely be wrong if you do. In most states, when there has been a transfer of funds and/or property to anyone within thirty to sixty months prior to the parent going into a nursing home, a client can be sanctioned for the transfer, which means you are guilty of a federal violation and must turn the funds over to Medicaid.

An estate plan is essential for people who want to protect their estate from recovery by Medicaid. We suggest you seek professional advice about estate plans. Most states have a mandate to recover funds in certain circumstances. However, the laws differ from state to state on this issue because Medicaid, a welfare program, is controlled by the state. In Utah, Medicaid will attempt recovery from the estate of a deceased individual who had received Medicaid assistance after age 55 and who has neither a surviving spouse nor a 100 percent disabled child. The Office of Recovery Services asserts a lien against the individual's home to recover any amount paid by Medicaid on a client's behalf. Medicaid is repaid from the value of this property.

When Mom died, Medicaid placed a lien on her home to recover funds it paid providers on her behalf. There are some exemptions. For example, if a Medicaid recipient has a dependent relative such as a daughter or grandson living in the same house to care for the elderly person, the relative can continue to live at the residence once the parent has died and efforts to recover funds will be forgiven. In this situation it is necessary to prove that the relative actually lived at the home for two years and was the dominant factor in keeping the elderly person out of a nursing home. Proof can take the form of a letter from the parent's physician verifying this state of affairs.

Some people accumulate substantial assets over the years so they can retire and live in comfort. When and if they become disabled, perhaps by a stroke or heart attack, they find they need special care. Living in a nursing care facility over a one-year period can cost well beyond $40,000, draining a person's life savings in a hurry. Once everything has been liquidated and spent down, Medicaid will take over the nursing home payments.

Why Won't Mom Ask for Help?

None of our parents liked to ask for our help directly. Why did they all act this way? Could it be because of the cohort effect where people of the same age are often similar because they have had similar life-experiences? Older adults who lived through the Great Depression continue to obsess about turning off home lights and saving money. The opposite is true of younger people who often leave lights burning for security reasons. Different philosophies. Different times.

We are not sure if some of the consistent behaviors we observed in our parents were the result of a cohort effect or if all of our parents possessed the same personality with regards to certain situations. When we visited Mom, she mimicked what our fathers said, "While you are here, I'll let you" or "While your not doing anything, do this for me." They avoided expressions like, "Would you do this for me?" or "Can you take me?" Each of our parents avoided directly asking for help: they gave subtle and sometimes not so subtle commands. Were these behaviors similar because of a cohort effect, a basic sense of pride, still wanting to "parent" a child or manipulative personalities?

We could have gotten caught in unpleasant exchanges with our parents if we didn't know the source of their commands. For example, when we told Mom we were unable to take her somewhere because of a prior commitment, she tried to lay a guilt trip on us by saying something like, "You never have time to do anything I want done or need to do" or "You never do anything I would like you to do." We said, "That's not true, we do a lot for you." Mom responded, " I've never asked you for anything." We started paying attention to how she worded her requests. We realized that in her mind, she was right—she never directly asked for anything. At first the way she tried to verbally manipulate us was upsetting. In retrospect, we realized her behavior was the same as our fathers. We just chuckled and continued to do what we could when we could, guilt free.

A large segment of the older population only know how to get what they want through making you feel guilty. This particular segment has never experienced how to give love—how to hug or kiss or say thank you. Psychologists call this guilt tripping by a professional. When faced with a parent behaving this way, do not be argumentative, it will only upset you and accomplish nothing. Use humor, it will help, as it did for me, when Mom said she had never asked us for anything. I responded with, "Sure, I've been taking you to the Friday night dance for the past twenty years because I love to dance, not because you do." She picked up on what I said and with both of us smiling, we dropped the issue. Even if Mom remembered a confrontation, it's rare she would mention it. While those we care for are sometimes reactive, they, like us, really don't want to create uncomfortable situations. We all had to learn how to let go of bad feelings and expectations.

Coping with Hearing Problems

Hearing impairment developed late in life can lead to social isolation but by seeking the aide of modern devices and positioning ourselves visibly for clear communication, the hearing impaired person can be helped. The tough part in convincing some people they need a hearing aid is that they hear so many negative things from former users.

Because she had no trouble hearing herself speak, Mom did not believe she had a hearing problem. However, she frequently responded to what she believed she heard, not to what was actually said. Still, it was impossible for us to convince her she had a hearing problem. We experienced a lot of frustration with her hearing impairment before we learned effective ways to communicate with her. Mom looked to us as interpreters by asking "What did he say?" She continually interrupted others with a topic of her own and usually people just stopped talking, let her speak, and then resumed their conversation as if Mom was not with the program.

Mom's hearing problem had quite an impact on her life. She became increasingly socially isolated when surrounded by people who found it easier to do things for her rather than just visit. She stopped asking family and friends to repeat themselves and pretty much remained silent.

We encouraged Mom to see an Otolaryngologist (ears, nose and throat physician) and have him test her for hearing impairment. We also offered to show a video featuring C. Everett Koop, MD, titled "Getting The Most Out Of Your Hearing Aids." Dr. Koop discusses the shoulds and should nots one can expect from hearing aids, the two types of hearing loss and how hearing aids can help. We tried to be positive in our presentation to her about wearing a hearing aid; however, Mom was not mentally ready to wear one. Because she was adamant about not wearing a hearing aid, which was the real issue, we stopped bringing up the subject. Since she would not wear one, we learned to adjust our forms of communication with her to account for her hearing loss.

When speaking to hearing impaired people, face them directly and make sure you have their attention before you speak. Don't speak with your hands covering your mouth or as you turn to leave a room. Keep out of shadows and speak clearly, slowly, naturally. Do not exaggerate lip movement. Avoid major conversations while driving because your lips are not easily visible. Alert others to these tips so they can converse with your parent without needing an interpreter.

Privacy versus Dangerous Secrets

Many elderly people do not believe they are vulnerable to outside influences and may, in their loneliness and desire for companionship, lose perspective on the dangers of today's society. They put themselves in great jeopardy when they allow the wrong people into their homes. We were always stressing the importance of not opening doors to strangers.

Mom, like many of her older friends, believed it was cute to be secretive and while their secrets were probably harmless, it only takes one to make a difference. I learned about one of Mom's harmless secrets when she and I were out driving, looking for somewhere to go and something to do. Since Snowbird resort was holding their annual Octoberfest, and the resort is located in one of Utah's most beautiful canyons, we decided to go there.

At Snowbird, Mom and I ran into John, a ninety-two-year-old friend. We were discussing the seniors citizen's dance where the two had originally met, when John asked, "Did your mother tell you about the motorcycle ride we took this past weekend to Kamas, Utah?" Mom tried to interrupt by changing the subject, but I persisted with "no, tell me about it." When John asked if it was OK, Mom told him to do whatever he wanted. She was upset and actually hoped he would just shut up. But he went ahead and told me the two had ridden his motorcycle approximately 100 miles round trip from Salt Lake City to Kamas.

Mom would never have told me about her cross country ride because she would have thought it was none of my business. This was exactly what she said when I asked. Although I was a little bit concerned about my 82-year-old mother burning rubber across the state with a 92-year-old motorcycle enthusiast, my fears were kept in check because she had known John for many years. This secret was more like an adventure than a potentially dangerous situation.

What I think of as a potentially dangerous situation for Mom began on a Saturday morning when she called, asking if I had felt the earthquake the night before. She had been sound asleep when her house suddenly begun to shake, and she awakened to a loud, banging noise and the sound of breaking glass. Since she had been too frightened to get out of bed, she waited until morning and that's when she found her broken hutch, glass vases, pictures and small trinkets spread all over the living room floor. Mom was trying to convince me there had been an earthquake and I didn't know why!

I drove to her house and was surprised to find the living room a disaster. Broken glass and pictures were scattered all over the room. Her china hutch had fallen over. I knew the hutch didn't fall due to an earthquake because the living room wreckage was restricted to just the hutch.

I told Mom I didn't believe her story about an earthquake. I told her I was going to call the University of Utah Seismograph station and see what areas had been affected. She said, "Fine," but when I called I was assured the Earth had not shook the night before. I told Mom I thought it odd that she wanted me to believe there was an earthquake. Angrily, she said she wasn't going to argue about it so the subject was dropped—for then. I cleaned up the mess and drove home.

A week later, as I entered Mom's home, I was again surprised, this time to discover a strange man noticeably younger than Mom sitting in her living room. He introduced himself to me and said he had met Mom the week before at the Friday senior's dance. This story seemed true enough. Mom had called us to say we didn't need to pick her up because a friend at the dance offered to give her a ride home. After the dance Mom and her new friend had breakfast and since it had been so late when he brought her home, Mom let him sleep on the couch. Around 2:00 a.m. he had to use the bathroom. When he got up from the couch, he tripped in the dark, grabbed the hutch and pulled it over. Mystery solved.

I told Mom it was dangerous to bring home someone she had just met and allow him to stay overnight. Sexual drives do not just stop one day. It was possible that he had been looking for her bedroom instead of the bathroom and maybe, had he found her, bad things would have happened and no one would have ever known he was there. Her response was, "It isn't any of your business."

Mom remained very independent in her thinking and we remained very cautious about what she told us. She didn't see people as threats to her life, but as conversation and company.

Since women outlive men approximately seven years, they look for companionship with vigor, sometimes placing themselves in an unpredictable situation. When transporting parents to a social function, let them know you worry about them and you don't want them to leave with anyone without notifying you first. If they do leave, make sure they tell someone you know.

Each parent's behavior is different; know yours and respond accordingly. The loss of a spouse, friend and family can create an unbearable loneliness which could lead someone to turn to strangers for companionship. Don't limit your parent's exposure to social acquaintances but do look out for them.

Creatures of Habit

We are all, to some extent, creatures of habit. Who doesn't have a familiar routine, cherished possession or a favorite way of doing things? Habits help us feel relaxed, secure and in control of our lives. For people who are forced to face drastic changes, such as the death of friends or loved ones and their own declining strength and health, keeping some things the same can be especially important.

Each parent has his or her own way of doing things. For example, when my father moved to Salt Lake City to live with us, bringing his collection of railroad memorabilia with him created a reassuring atmosphere in his new surroundings, and helped him hang onto his sense of who he was. When Emily's father had setbacks in his health, we would always emphasize to him the goal of getting back to his routine. Even though it would have been very boring for us—doing, even eating, exactly the same things every day—it gave him a sense of security and independence.

Mom's habits and routines were also very important to her. She never got up before 10 a.m. and always had coffee and toast for breakfast. The dishes were washed and replaced in the cupboard right after the meal was finished. She smoked excessively in her later years and made those around her nervous many times because she threw her cigarette butts into a paper bag before the cigarette was out, leaving the potential for a fire. She turned the television on for the four o'clock news and left it on until two in the morning. And because she had a hearing problem, she kept the volume up. Her house was always tidy.

Mom was able to care for herself in her own home, but there were still times when we disrupted her habits by trying to do something for her that she was not happy with us doing. We learned the importance of avoiding disruptive changes in her life whenever possible, while at the same time keeping in mind some changes might actually make her life easier and more enjoyable in the long run.

Your parents may not always appreciate the effort you go to in helping them maintain old habits or establish new ones. Cope with catering to their desires by setting reasonable limits while never neglecting their urgent needs. When it appears they don't appreciate how hard you work to help them maintain a quality life, remind yourselves that their attitudes are a reflection of the amount of stress they feel when their lives are disrupted rather than an indication of how they feel about you.

Mom's Appliance Woes

Sometimes it seems like everybody in America is ready to sell you something "new and improved." When it comes to our parents though, "old and familiar" might be a better slogan. Unfortunately, it took us more than one "lesson" to learn Mom did not always want something "new" when she said she did.

In 1947, my parents purchased a kitchen stove. Then one day in 1993, Mom called to inform us that her oven was no longer working. She needed a new one and wanted me to choose it. I told her I'd rather take her somewhere so she could select the one she wanted. So we went shopping.

Mom was disappointed to discover that all new stoves had limited storage space and most had digital dials. However, after looking at the styles and her options, she finally picked one and made arrangements for delivery. Mom called a friend who owns a four-apartment complex and told him he could have her old stove, but the oven needed to be repaired. He agreed to pick it up the same day her new one was delivered.

From day one, Mom never stopped complaining about her new stove. She didn't like the digital controls behind the burners because when she reached to turn the controls off, she burned her arm. She soon told me she had contacted her friend and asked if he would return her old stove, now repaired, in exchange for her new $640 stove. He was happy to make the exchange. It would have been easier, cheaper and made Mom happier, if we had just fixed her old stove.

A similar situation happened with the refrigerator she and my father had purchased in 1947. After that trusty old refrigerator broke down, Mom would have been perfectly happy if we had repaired it but unfortunately, we did what she said she wanted—we purchased a new frig and again she never stopped complaining. Thereafter, whenever a repairman told us it will cost $200 or more to repair a parent's forty- or fifty-year-old appliance, we told them to FIX IT!

When looking for a replacement of an appliance that can't be repaired, you could have a similar experience to our outing when Mom's vacuum stopped working. She wanted one like her fifty-year-old torpedo-shaped vacuum—small, light weight with a very long extension hose. Since it was beyond repair and we couldn't find anything comparable, we thought she might like one like ours. But after considering our options and remembering the lesson we had learned, we decided to wait. This was a good decision. We had practically exhausted the search of appliance stores when we finally found a similar vacuum. Amazingly, Mom thought it was perfect because it was so similar to her old one.

If you can fix something, fix it; however, if it can't be repaired, thoroughly investigate what your parent really wants before purchasing anything. Will the appliance controls and digital dials be too complex? Where are the controls positioned? What color is best and what size? Will it store as much stuff as the old appliance? If you don't assume, you will save time, energy and frustration.

When New is an Improvement and When it's Not

When aged parents ask their adult children to make a major purchase, it is important that the specifics are understood. Do your parents desire a new stove because they want to modernize the home or is it because the old one needs repairs? If they know it can be repaired, and still want a new one, ask why. Will they understand the new technology that manufacturers are building into their products? How can you determine, when discussing new features that make life easier, if they really mean no when they say yes?

If Mom didn't have a television, her daily routine of watching it would be disrupted so when her TV quit working, knowing the urgency of finding another, we embarked on another appliance hunt. It was the same experience, new area—electronics.

Mom's old remote control had a simple on/off button, an up/down channel button, an up/down sound button and a color button. But when she purchased one with a wider range of functions on the remote she thought she would like it better. There were push buttons for power, cable, VCR, TV, closed caption, flashback, mute, channel, volume, enter, menu, quit, record, pause, timer, TV/VCR source, rewind, color, play, stop and fast forward. Once at home, the reality was she was overwhelmed *and* confused. One day she called and asked if I could come to her home and fix the color on her television; it was too red. We found she had accidentally pushed the color button on her remote control, adding too much red. Sometime later, she called because she couldn't get sound: unknowingly she had pushed her mute button. Next, she had sound, but no picture: she pushed the VCR button which converted the TV to the VCR. We pushed the same button and it switched back. We soon started to direct her over the telephone to push the power button on the television, turning it off then on again, resetting the features on the television in the process. "Voila," the picture would reappear.

Mom's problem was with the overwhelming array of buttons, not the television. The new fangled remote controls did not make her life easier. In fact, they made all our lives a bit more unpleasant. Does this mean all so-called improvements will backfire? Not necessarily. A microwave oven is a sophisticated piece of technology but Mom loved the one we gave her, because it was easy to use. She merely pushed a button and out popped the door. She turned the single dial left for defrost, or right for cooking. When she turned the timer-dial right and closed the door, it started cooking for the number of minutes she had set on the timer. We found new appliances could help Mom maintain her independence if she readily understood how they worked. The key to getting her the microwave oven was to stay away from the digital programming kind and keep it simple. Now does this mean all elderly people have the same difficulties as Mom? Of course not. But our solutions may be beneficial for caregivers who experience what we did.

If manufacturers would offer a simple remote control with only on-off, volume and sound buttons, most anyone could operate it. If someone is confused with how to operate an appliance that item will either collect dust or create plenty of inconvenience for everyone. Remember, what you find useful and enjoyable might be frustrating for someone else.

Are We Helping or Interfering?

It can be difficult discerning what might be helpful from what might cause frustration. Making changes in a parent's home, yard, furniture, appliances and so on can make them either happy or upset. It would be a mistake to make any change that would unnecessarily disrupt or alter their life style, especially if they are perfectly happy with the way things are. Even when a parent seems to appreciate what you are about to do, you may face disapproval and dissatisfaction during the process.

After I removed Mom's lawn mower, the only thing she needed to do was water, but watering became increasingly difficult and her lawn was starting to turn brown. A friend of mine volunteered to assist me in putting an automatic sprinkler system in Mom's yard. Since he was a student, we needed to work around his time schedule. He estimated two weeks to complete the job. Mom would come outside everyday and complain about the holes, trenches, pipes, tools and dirt scattered throughout her yard. She only saw the mess, not the finished product, and was not a happy camper. It wasn't until we finished installation, had everything buried, her yard cleared of equipment and supplies, that she finally calmed down. Even though she was stressed out for two weeks, I think, in the long run, Mom would have been even more stressed had her entire yard turned brown.

One day, Emily and I went to an open house next door to Mom's house. The floor plan was identical to hers, except for a breakfast bar that had been built where the kitchen wall once stood: adding personality and increasing space. We described to Mom what her neighbor's kitchen and living room looked like but because she was perfectly happy with hers the way it was, we did nothing. It would have been a mistake to make changes in her home she didn't want because it would have only caused her frustration and mental anguish. Because of her response to change, we began to refrain from instigating additional improvements.

Before making any changes to a parent's home, first have their approval. Then before acting, weigh all options. Take nothing for granted! When people age, they don't want change, they want uniformity and familiarity.

The Dangers of Combining Medications

It is not unusual for people to develop health problems as a result of taking dangerous combinations of otherwise safe medications. There are certain contributing factors that can lead to this. We have known elderly people who save, trade and then take, medication with no idea of what interaction will take place when combining prescriptions. They remove medication from one container and place it in another without changing labels, then some time later, forgetting the change, take something totally different than what was in the original container. Expiration dates mean nothing to many of the elderly. Those who do not live under the watchful eye of a caregiver may mix old medicine with new, putting themselves in harm's way.

For these reasons, it is important to have some control over when and what medications a parent takes. Assemble all medications, then read each label for it's medical name, use, expiration date and dosage. Flush expired medicine down the toilet. Encourage your doctor to write on all prescriptions what the medication is for so the pharmacist can, in turn, give you better information. Compare the dosage instructions you received from the doctor with what the pharmacist writes on the label to determine if the doctor's handwriting was read correctly.

If you purchase all medications from one pharmacy, you will have one record at one location. You can easily inform the pharmacists and the physician of all medications being taken, even those prescribed by other physicians, so they will be alert to potential interactions. When helping your parent take oral medication, know what is being taken.

Do not assume that taking medication is a simple task for your older parents. We left our parents alone with their medication in a one inch diameter paper cup and a glass of water with the assumption they would take their pills. Occasionally, when we returned, there would be a pill lying on a lap, on the floor or in the cup. So we began to observe pill taking so we could be of assistance when necessary. If a parent refused to take medication, we explained the possible consequences of sickness or death, then encouraged them to take the pill. We didn't support decisions not to take medication, but it was their right to make that choice.

Many people are not aware that aspirin and Advil, taken together, can be dangerous. How dangerous? On April 30, 1994, Mom called. I could hardly hear what she was saying. I did hear, "I need help" and I responded with, "I'm on my way." As soon as we disconnected, I dialed 911 and told the operator that my 85-year-old mother had just called and needed help. I gave her mother's name, address and phone number, and told her I would meet the paramedics at Mom's house.

Mom had her screen doors locked when the paramedics arrived and since they won't break and enter unless absolutely necessary, they waited for me. They could see Mom through the screen door, sitting in a chair next to her telephone and even though she appeared to be semi-conscious, she was unable to stand or speak. I punched a hole in the screen, unhooked the latch and let the paramedics in. They immediately checked her vitals. They couldn't find a pulse or blood pressure so they took her to the hospital. It was amazing she had been able to dial our telephone number for help.

I called Mom's doctor and she had Mom admitted to the hospital. She ordered some tests run so she could formulate an idea as to what may be going on. Mom was admitted with a diagnosis of upper gastrointestinal bleeding. Upon admittance, she was stabilized by the transfusion of three units of packed, red blood cells. She was given two more units of blood that evening. Another doctor was brought in to act as a consultant and he proceeded to follow her closely throughout her hospital stay in case surgical intervention was needed. Later on, judging from her blood count, blood pressure and pulse, the doctor was confident that Mom had stabilized and considered her fit for discharge by the morning of May 7, 1994.

Mom was discharged to our home where we could closely supervise her recovery. Professional Nursing Services evaluated her and the clinical findings showed a decrease in balance and a tendency to fall to her right. She had poor posture and needed standby assistance for showering, walking and climbing stairs. An aide, therapist and nurse came to our home weekly to assist with her daily living activities.

The doctor told us the reason Mom had developed a large ulcer was that she had been taking aspirin daily to reduce the risk of having a stroke. Unknown to us, she also had been taking Advil daily for headaches. Together, the two chemically burned a huge hole in the upper part of Mom's small intestine called a duodenal ulcer. This combination, appearing harmless to Mom, caused a frightening and painful condition. We reiterate the importance of knowing exactly what medications are being taken.

Getting Mom Back to Her Routines

Our goal, getting Mom back in her home, would take approximately six weeks to accomplish. It was necessary for the three of us to understand what expectations we had of one another while living together. We felt it necessary to set guidelines, even for a short stay. When people, who have been hospitalized or placed in a nursing home, know they will eventually return to their own home, their attitude is different from individuals who know they will never return. Emily and I again confirmed this when the two of us went to Mom's hospital room, just before she was to be discharged.

Mom knew she was being discharged to our home where the two of us could supervise her recovery over the four to six weeks of therapy she needed to regain her strength before returning to her own home. We told her if she needed privacy, she could go to the sanctuary of her bedroom, where she would have her own telephone and television. No one would enter her room without permission and we would help with whatever she needed but only until her strength returned. We didn't eat at any particular time, but would prepare whatever foods she enjoyed and she could eat whenever and wherever she wanted. We noticed the foods she wanted were foods she did not normally prepare for herself, things that she had forgotten how to prepare like poached eggs and pancakes for breakfast. This gave us more insight into what she had given up in her life in order to continue to stay in her own home.

On occasion, Mom would insist on washing dishes, and when she did, because of poor eyesight, the dishes were never clean. Since we were going to wash them in the first place, rather than pointing out that they were still dirty, we would simply wash them again, not saying anything and leaving her with a sense of accomplishment and contribution. It also alerted us to the fact that she needed more assistance with the upkeep of her home.

When we first brought Mom to our home, she really liked the attention and she would express her appreciation for all the things we were doing. Nevertheless, during the six weeks she was with us, Mom went from a weak, frail, little old lady, to an argumentative and demanding old woman. Nothing pleased her. She tried to change our lifestyle to hers, something we would not let happen. She was antsy to return home. Because she was functioning much better, we knew it was time.

We conferred with the nurse and she agreed that Mom was physically ready to return home. We gathered up her belongings and in a couple of days drove her back home where she could return to her daily routines.

Once we were aware of a potential danger (in Mom's case, the stairs to her basement laundry room), it was necessary to intervene to ensure there would be no accidents. The day she returned home, we suggested that, for safety reasons, we do her laundry. Thereafter, every other Friday, we picked up her laundry and returned it the next day.

From the day she was admitted into the hospital for her ulcer, our mutual goal was to get Mom back home as soon as possible. For over two years after she returned to her home, she was able to keep her Friday schedule of shopping, getting her hair done and going to the dance at the senior citizen's complex. The only changes made in her routines were that we did her laundry and a housekeeper cleaned and sanitized her kitchen and bathroom weekly. At first it was hard for her to accept the housekeeper, but gradually, as she found things more difficult to do, she was pleased to have the service and the company.

Mom's change in personality while living with us was characteristic of a pattern of personality change in elderly women. Women who have always been the obedient, nurturing peacemakers throughout their younger years tend to turn aggressive and argumentative in their older years.

An opposite change in behavior is characteristic of men. Those men who were controlling, aggressive and, perhaps, abusive throughout their younger years, tend to become, for the most part, docile and easy going in their later years. Unfortunately, because of this reversal in behavior, it is easier for the caregiver to work through a forgiveness process with the men by caring for the now, mild-mannered person, than it is to remember the once caring, gentle arms of a now bitter and angry old woman. Knowing that this personality change is so common helped us to have patience with Mom when she was in a particularly difficult mood.

Mom Comes to Garfield Avenue

Emily and I have stated many times that we utilized the time our parent's were hospitalized or rehabilitating in a nursing home to determine what will be needed once they are released. Before being released, taking a parent to their home and allowing them freedom to move about will help you decide whether your parent can live alone. You can see, first hand, whether they will ignore or forget what hospital and nursing home staff have told them. Also you will see whether they are disoriented and confused in old familiar surroundings.

Until Mom's fall November 23, 1996, when she sustained compressed fractures of four vertebrae, she did a good job of caring for herself. Because of her injury, she was hospitalized for approximately two weeks, then spent an additional three weeks rehabilitating in a nursing home. On Christmas day Emily and I thought we might get lucky once again, as we were with my father: when we took him home from the nursing home in Ohio Thanksgiving day a few years ago, he had functioned so well. We took Mom home Christmas to see how she would get along in familiar surroundings, but she was disoriented and extremely confused in her own home. We were there only minutes when Mom wanted to show us she could walk without her walker, something her therapist didn't want Mom to do. Mom got up and walked to her bedroom and, unknown to her, I was close behind. Mom turned, lost her balance and fell. I caught her. She walked to the living room and again she fell. I caught her. When I tried to explain to her that we thought it best she come live with us because she had fallen twice in a matter of minutes, she denied she had ever fallen. In her mind she was right: because I caught her, she had not fallen.

As we continued to watch her throughout the afternoon, Mom appeared to have difficulty using the telephone. Thinking I understood her problem, I explained that she couldn't just hold the receiver while deciding what number to dial, she needed to lift the receiver and dial immediately. After a few minutes of explanation, I realized she thought the telephone was the TV controls and she was actually trying to turn the TV on. After an exhausting day of confusion, Emily and I, as well as Mom, knew she would not be able to live by herself. Later that evening we returned her to the nursing home and began preparation to bring her home with us.

When we returned from Dad's Kentucky burial on Saturday, December 28, we spoke with Mom in the nursing home. We told her we couldn't afford to pay someone to live with her around the clock, that few people would be willing to stay with her in exchange for room and board. Potential caregivers would probably also be put off by her smoking habit and playing the television late at night. It was evident the nursing home had made a lasting impression with Mom, evident by her stating over and over that she wanted to leave there and come live with us. She did not want to be restricted to a semi-private room with a sick elderly stranger for a roommate. She did not want to be put to bed each night, by seven p.m. or made to eat breakfast by six a.m. Since she agreed to work with us, we moved her in to our home the following day.

We mentioned earlier that when people know they will eventually return to their own home, their attitude is different from someone who knows they will never return from nursing home placement. The last time Mom stayed with us, she knew she would return to her home; her personality changed in six short weeks. But when she knew she would never return to her home, she was very adaptable and pleasant.

Because Mom needed physical therapy and assistance with bathing, we decided to try a different home health agency from the one Dad used. The difference was amazing. While Dad's aide had been terrific, everyone in the new agency, the nurse, physical therapist and aides were dedicated, thorough and hard working professionals. At no time did we feel slighted in the care given. This was our first positive experience with a home health physical therapist. He spent a full half hour working vigorously with Mom and when through, Mom knew she had had a workout. The nurse showed great compassion and never hurried when she interviewed Mom. These professionals are what home health care is all about and why things work in home caregiving.

With the assistance of our home health agency, we intended to care for Mom for the rest of her life. This was to be a short lived commitment. After living with us for only nineteen days, Mom, like our fathers, waited until we were by her side before she died peacefully in our home on Garfield Avenue.

Taken by Surprise and Then There were None

Mom seemed to be adjusting well to her surroundings and, after two weeks of hard work, her physical therapist had helped her manage her walker where we felt comfortable leaving her alone for an hour or so. On January 16, Mom requested we go to her home to fetch some clothes she wanted and as we were leaving she commented on how good a bologna sandwich was I had fixed for her; these were to be her last words to me.

Mom had pretty much settled into her routines in her new home. At four o'clock in the afternoon she turned on the television. At four thirty she turned the light on next to her chair. On the day we went to fetch her clothes, we returned at ten minutes after five and found Mom sitting in her chair, slumped slightly to one side; she was unconscious but alive. We took her hand in ours and told her we were with her and we would take care of her. Emily went quickly to the phone and called our home health nurse and reported what we found, a hospice nurse was alerted and dispatched to our home. As Emily talked to the nurse, I told Mom I loved her. Mom's shoulders sort of hunched and through pursed lips she slightly jerked forward forcing out air. I repeated, "I love you Mom" and she did exactly the same thing. I told Emily to come in because I felt Mom was going fast and I wanted both of us to be with her when she died. When Emily came in she took Mom's hand and for the last time I wanted to see if Mom would react as before. I said "I love you, Mom" and she did. In my heart, I know she heard me. Emily said, "You can let go now, Mom" and I repeated "You can let go now, Mom." And she did.

Celebrating the Life of a Free Spirit

Mom never said where her parents were buried. She had no family ties and never mentioned wanting to be buried anywhere specific. Mom was a free spirit of her own. She was as independent in her dying as she was in her living. Death was something she didn't like to discuss; as she would say, "You live until you die and then you die, that's it."

Mom didn't have a pre-paid burial plan; she wanted Byron and me to do with her as we thought best. Rather than have a viewing or graveside services Byron and I decided to use the obituaries to invite friends and relatives to come to our home to celebrate Mom's life. We had an excellent turnout of relatives, old friends and neighbors from years past who wanted to participate in Mom's celebration. All of her life Mom never saw herself as anyone other than the vibrant 18-year-old girl she once was so we placed youthful pictures of her throughout our living and dining room, showing her free spirit when around people she enjoyed. Everyone had stories to tell about how Mom influenced their lives and all appeared to have a good time.

Since Mom had no preference to what we should do with her body, we believed Mom's free spirit would agree to crema tion. The day after our celebration for Mom, Emily and I brought home a gray plastic box wrapped in blue paper. The box weighed five pounds and contained a clear plastic bag with Mom's ashes. Mom looked like dried sand on a California beach. For the first time since her death, I felt good holding what was once the shell that housed the spirit of my mother.

The realism that all of our parents are now dead and buried leaves us reflective and with a daily void. While we will miss them all, we know they are now free.

One More Lesson: Estate Sales

If you must liquidate a household, do so when you are emotionally able to deal with shallow people.

Mother left her home and furniture to Byron and me. We had decisions to make about the house: to rent her home, repairs would be minimal; to sell it, remodeling could be substantial. Before these decisions could be made we had to probate Mom's will. Since she had no estate we first needed to probate her will through the courts which could take up to six months. To probate means to 1. prove that a will is valid; 2. identify the personal representative or representatives who will execute the requests made in the will; and 3. establish the deceased person had no financial obligations.

Once the will was probated, Byron and I boxed up the things we wanted from the home. Then we prepared for an estate sale to liquidate the balance. Because we were novices in the business of selling estates, we went to several sales and asked questions. We were advised, for example, to hire a professional appraiser and not divulge we were having an estate sale, but to say pricing was needed for insurance purposes. Good advice. If not, we were cautioned the appraiser could price items high, only to return and purchase at half price what was not sold in the sale.

Despite our "field research," our estate sale was a nightmare. Once our ad ran in the local paper we were worked by dealers and professional shoppers. People hounded us in person and by phone, day and night, to examine items before the sale. People pretentiously offered help before the sale by insisting that if we let them in before the sale they could give us valuable pricing information that would help us. They suggested we just let five or six people in at the same time. They informed us of the difficulty in controlling crowds, when in fact they and their friends were the first five or six people in line — with boxes.

Once we let people in on the day of the sale, they were like vultures stuffing their boxes with collectible items. They broke and stole things and had a complete disregard for our home and our loss. It was difficult seeing what represented Mom's life for so many years being fragmented by such insensitive gluttons. Eventually I had to ask people to leave.

In retrospect we wonder if we placed a large picture of Mom on the wall with a sign saying, "The Estate of Hazel Watson," would its presence have jarred the heads of this unthinking segment. Would they have shown more respect.

Since we will not have the opportunity to test this theory, if any of you experiment with it or other ideas, let us know about your results. We also would love to hear of solutions you have discovered in your caregiving roles. Write to:

People Helping People Maintain Dignity
PMD Vision
P. O. Box 520157
Salt Lake City UT 84152
E-mail: gew@call-pmd.com
http://www.call-pmd.com

Amen, Amen, I say to you
when you were younger, you used to dress yourself
and go where you wanted; but when you grow old
you will stretch out your hands and someone else will
dress you and lead you where you do not want to go.

John 21:18

CONTINUUM

Throughout the ages caring for those who have given us life and then grown old has been a well traveled path. It is a path that will continue to be traveled, not just by those of you currently on it, but also by the children who will follow you. The experiences we have shared with you were expressed in the hopes you realize you are not alone as you face this challenge of parent care. We have presented situations in detail throughout the book to impress upon you the amount of energy and time required should you chose to meet the challenge. We have also provided you with lessons we've learned both through these experiences and through our formal education to assist with insurance, Medicare and community services.

What we want to close with is the understanding that the chores we did and the sacrifices we made cannot be measured against the rewards we have both experienced, rewards such as having both of our fathers finally referring to our house as their home. We had the pleasure of creating a high trust level concerning their health care. We experienced the joy of hearing not only our fathers' but our mother's laugh and seeing them smile while engaged in conversation. We sensed that our touch, our back rubs and foot rubs, relaxed them when they ached physically or emotionally. We learned low, gentle talking would ease their confusion.

We improved our relationship with our parents and put unfinished business to rest. Seeing these very special people through a vulnerable stage of their life, all the way to death's door, was our final gift to them. Doing what you can for as long as you can could be your final gift to your parents.

As you face THE CALLING, the challenge of caring for your parents, may you and your loved ones experience the dignity and feel the inner consolation that comes when a path is traveled in communion.

INDEX